Bodycraft

Bodycraft

Creating the Body You Want
While Loving the Body You Have

L. Ilizabethe Zélandais

ANTI-GRAVITY PRESS
SACRAMENTO, CALIFORNIA

Bodycraft: Creating the Body You Want While Loving the Body You Have.

Publisher's Note:
The author of this book does not prescribe any technique as treatment for physical, medical, emotional or mental problems without the advice of a professional practioner. The author and publisher expressly disclaim responsibility for liability, loss or risk, personal or otherwise, which is incurred as a consequence, directly or indirectly, of the use and application of any of the contents of this book. If you choose to use this information, the author and publisher assume no responsibility for your actions.

Cataloging-in-Publication Data
Zélandais, L. Ilizabethe.
    Bodycraft : creating the body you want while loving the body you have / L. Ilizabethe Zélandais.
    p. cm.
    Includes bibliographical references.
    LCCN 94-76849
    ISBN 0-9640961-0-2

    1. Body image.   2. Physical fitness.   I. Title

BF697.5.S43Z45 1994   158'.1
                                           QBI94-970

To my daughter, Carrie Prehoda.
You bring light and lightness to every situation.

Table of Contents

Acknowledgements

Gratitude is the memory of the heart.
-Herbert V. Prochnow

I would like to express my gratitude and mention by name the many professionals who gave generously of their time, expertise and encouragement in the writing of this book. William A. Tiller, Professor Emeritus, Department of Materials Science and Engineering of Stanford University shared his research regarding the effects of focused human attention. Dr. Jack Holland of the Institute for Human Growth and Awareness has been an inspiration with his integrative work in science and spirituality, and he also kindly put me in touch with Dr. Tiller. Dr. Larry Dossey (a seeker of truth in his ongoing investigation of science, medicine and prayer) helped me track down Spindrift, Inc. Dr. Leroy R. Perry, Jr., Olympic Sports chiropractor and president of the International Sportsmedicine Institute of Los Angeles, provided invaluable information about the importance of water in the diet. The American Physical Therapy Association graciously allowed me to reprint excerpts from their excellent brochure on posture. Any error in facts in no way reflects on any of these fine professionals, but rather on my interpretation.

My thanks goes to these individuals for reading the manuscript and offering many helpful comments:

> Debra Barbour
> Teri Callaghan
> Nancy Jongeward, MFCC
> Randal Posey, M.D.
> Nancy Widby

I extend my appreciation to Dave Barry's agent, A. L. Hart of The Fox Chase Agency, Inc., who stated, "We regret that we feel we cannot grant permission for you to quote the Dave Barry material cited in your letter." I regret that they feel that way, too, because it was a great quote about bathroom scales. I would nevertheless like to thank them for replying so promptly and for making me aware that there are actually agents who have feelings.

I would like to thank my ex-husband Gary Prehoda for encouraging me to write long before I was willing to do it.

And thank *you*, for reading my book, stimulating the economy, and being good to yourself. Although I may not know you personally, I have known that you are there. Without you, *BODYCRAFT* never would have happened.

❦

Preface

Destiny is not a matter of chance, it is a matter of choice; it is not a thing to be waited for, it is a thing to be achieved.

-William Jennings Bryan

I am now a winner every day of my life, and this book is a result of my winning experience. That experience includes overcoming years of overweight, food disorders and yo-yo dieting. The first question most people ask is what I had to give up.

First, I had to give up not being a winner. I had to accept being a winner no matter what I looked like, no matter what the scales said or, most of all, no matter what anybody else said or thought about me. Next, I gave up overweight, food disorders and yo-yo dieting.

From my earliest memories, food was the central focus in our home. As Depression survivors, my parents viewed keeping their family well-fed as the ultimate demonstration of their love, and I learned to feed myself altogether too well.

Throughout my school years, I felt trapped in a body always bigger than any of the "cute girls". Wanting to fit in, I began the years of dieting—see-sawing from the ecstasy of acceptable thinness to the shame of being once more overcome by a sugary binge. The scales became my best enemy, especially after one particularly "successful" diet.

As a college junior, I had just proudly dieted my 5'8" frame down to 120 pounds and a Size 6 dress. Suddenly, horribly I started craving sweets and could not stop eating them (in retrospect a natural physical response to what the body recognizes as starvation). Even as I could not resist all I had been denying myself, neither could I stand the idea of losing my slender body. Thus began the binge and purge cycle of bulimia.

This was in 1973 when "food disorder" was not a household word. I felt isolated, alone and constantly fearful of someone finding out this shameful secret.

I eventually tamed the vicious cycle to only occasional occurrences, and I also returned to being fat. Weight and food continued to be obsessions as I pursued every avenue promising the miracle of thinness. The following years were marked by temporary successes predictably overcome by the compulsion to overeat.

Shortly after I became pregnant, I had one more bulimic experience; and this time I realized my shame was for what I might be doing to my baby. I never again binged or had another bulimic occurrence, but I was still consumed with the same issues of body and soul.

Even after Carrie was born, I was more absorbed by getting back into my jeans than by the love I could give to a brand new person. This is the worst part of any obsession/compulsion: it sidelines us from and robs us of Life.

I continued trying anything to be slender and stay that way, but somewhere along the path it became more of a commitment to fulfill all I could be. I accumulated tools and methods that supported me in every part of my life, and which also helped me overcome my food addiction. This became the basis for Bodycraft.

One day I realized I could eat one or two cookies and did not have to physically restrain myself to keep from eating the entire bag. I recognized a basic core of peace in my life, and it extended to my eating habits.

I can't say that I have arrived at some final destination of perfect control. Sometimes I still find myself standing in front of the refrigerator until my nose hairs ice over. I am still on the journey, but I have come to believe the statement, "The journey is the destination."

I haven't binged in over 15 years. My life is balanced, and above all, I'm happy. As a bonus, I have a slender, toned body that I feel great to be alive in!

Just as Bodycraft has changed my life and appearance, it can do the same for you.

❦

Chapter One

Bodycraft: A New Vision

There is no ultimate answer, but there is an ultimate question: "Can you live with it?"

Just as your life is shaped by your many different facets—physical, mental, emotional, and spiritual—so is your body. By nurturing these different levels, you can reshape yourself and your form.

You *can* create and craft your body to be the way you have always wanted it. That may sound like a futuristic myth, particularly if you have tried every diet and exercise program on the market, plus a few of your own. Why should this experience be any more successful, any less frustrating, any different than those you have already so painfully experienced?

The key difference is that Bodycraft works *with* you, rather than forcing you to struggle to be someone and something you're not. This process supports you and your needs of body, mind, spirit and emotions. Unlike many programs, Bodycraft does *not* view you as simply a body that only needs the willpower to eat less and exercise more.

You have undoubtedly been telling yourself in many different ways that you will be a winner and love yourself when . . . . Those messages may go something like:

"I will love myself (my body) when I look like a *Vogue* or *GQ* model."

"I will love myself when someone else loves me."

"I will. . . I will. . . I will. . . when. . . when. . . when. . ."

You may not consciously say those words, but the message is there loud and clear. Instead of achieving self-satisfaction and the vibrant body image you want, those messages weigh down both your self-esteem and your body.

How would you respond if your best friend looked at you and said, "You look absolutely awful! I won't have anything to do with you until you lose 15 pounds of ugly fat!"?

Pretty traumatic, huh? It's doubtful you would feel particularly motivated to do anything such a person might suggest even if those suggestions were in your best interests.

Yet how often do you treat yourself with such hateful lack of respect? How many critical, negative messages are you giving yourself daily or even hourly? Has it helped make any positive changes?

At this very moment you are a winner who is worthy of love simply because you are uniquely and beautifully you. The time to accept that and to love yourself is now. That may be a tall order to change the negative self-concepts, ugly messages and mean ways of treating yourself, but you can do it—and now is the time to start.

This is the first step in the journey of the proverbial thousand miles: making a conscious choice to love yourself *exactly as you are this moment* warts and all; deciding to treat yourself nicer than (or at least as nicely as) you treat anybody else; and resolving to give yourself only positive messages.

Paradoxically, loving yourself as you are now is the only key to lasting positive change later. Even if you manage to make the changes while promising to love yourself "when", you will still be holding the love carrot just slightly out of reach; and the *Vogue/GQ* body and the relationship still will not be enough.

This entire Bodycraft process is about wholeness. It is about caring for the wholeness of your body while paying attention to all the parts; and it is about wholeness as opposed to perfection. (Wherever the word "perfect" or its derivatives are used in this book, think of it as meaning "just right for me" or "exactly what I want".)

We usually flog ourselves with a goal of perfection corresponding to some ideal standard. Just whose ideal? And who wants to be standard, whatever that is? Wholeness is the integration and weaving of our strengths and limitations, our light sides and our dark sides, into a tapestry of beauty and texture.

This can be our highest goal for our bodies and our lives. I ask you to share that vision and goal for yourself as you learn the art of Bodycraft.

Chapter Two

Dump the Diet Habit Forever

*Principles have no real force except when
one is well fed.*

-Mark Twain

Of the 50 million Americans who annually attempt yet another weight-loss program, 98% do not experience long-term success. (And where are the 2% who do?)

In spite of such discouraging odds, these extreme regimens often seem to be the only alternatives to obesity. So the frustrated, discontented and disillusioned masses continue going on the latest greatest fad diets and "fat-burning" exercise programs. And even as they start another New Year's or another Monday with another diet, they know that there is a 98% chance they will be disappointed again.

When are they going to get it? By themselves THESE PROGRAMS DON'T WORK. Many of them completely

5

derail the metabolism, setting up the hopeful dieter to get fatter. But the reasons they don't work for the long haul go beyond even that sad news.

1. Diets do not support our motivations and needs.

Most diets address only the physical. What could be more pointless? If we ate only for physical reasons, there would be no market for diet books.

In truth, we eat because we are happy or sad. We eat because our parents made us clean our plates decades ago. We eat to celebrate. We eat to socialize. We eat to think more clearly. We eat in order not to think at all. We eat for religious holidays. We eat for secular holidays. We eat because it is not a holiday. Ad infinitum.

Nevertheless, diets—and the books and authors promoting them—continue to aim at only physical consumption. While we are already quite well-versed in taking care of our physical requirements, needs of the mind, emotions and soul are being overlooked.

2. Diets ask us to buy into deprivation.

The origin of the word "diet" comes from the Greek word meaning "manner of living". Yet today's concept of diet has degenerated to what most of us would inter- pret as "manner of the living dead". There are many excellent diets which support health and nutrition, but they nourish *only* the body while the soul is left to starve. It's time to get back to the original Greek view of what we eat as a part of the whole quality-of-life picture.

3. Diets put us down.

Most lose-weight, feel-the-burn, fix-your-body routines are alien to who and what we are designed to be. We end up fighting ourselves; and who ever won a shadowboxing match?

Rather than acknowledging we are perfect just as we are at this moment and helping us evolve from there, diet and exercise plans frequently promote a subtle message that we are not quite acceptable as we are. Their general tone implies that unless we perfectly follow the dictates of the current weight-loss program, we will continue to be unacceptable. None of us thrive and bloom and live happily for the long-term unless we are supported in being great for who and what we are at any given moment.

4. Diets do not help us adjust our self-perceptions as we adjust our bodies.

Sometimes people are actually successful through diet and exercise alone in creating the body they want. Unfortunately, it will never last if that person has not changed the inner perception of self.

Who we think and feel we are will always win out as a self-fulfilling prophecy. If we haven't translated our desired body image to the other parts of our self-concept—mental, emotional and spiritual—the physical body will spring back to the image we hold at our deepest levels.

None of this is meant to diminish the importance of the proper care and maintenance of our bodies through good nutrition and adequate physical activity. However, effective change must go far beyond slam-dunking ourselves into rigid and often stupid programs which guarantee only a loss of self-esteem.

5. Diets address the symptoms and not the cause.

The body is just one energy system giving us clues we are in balance and harmony. If your body and body image are not the reflection you desire, it is like the red lights on your car dashboard indicating an overheated motor or low oil.

Trying to change only your body is like trying to make your car's red warning lights go off without adjusting the underlying problem. There are any number of ways to deal with the warning lights; but if you do anything other than treating the difficulty they are indicating, your car problems are going to become increasingly severe.

Similarly, if you don't correct the imbalances of other systems your body monitors, you may manage to pound your outer form into shape, but you will continue to become more emotionally discontent, mentally stressed and spiritually out-of-step.

This book is about being or becoming a craftsperson who lovingly, gently, and non-intrusively molds and shapes your entire system back into balance; and it is about having a body which reflects that. It's okay if the body is your main goal—as a by-product, you get a balanced, harmonious self. These are all roads leading to the same place—and Bodycraft is the vehicle to take you there.

Chapter Three

What to Expect

To change one's life:
Start immediately.
Do it flamboyantly.
No exceptions.
        -William James

You are your own best authority, and Bodycraft is a personalized tool to fit your best interests. Unless you borrowed this book, write in it, dog-ear special pages, and slash through sections you may disagree with. Make it *your* tool by interpreting and using what suits you best.

The only way you can do this wrong is by ignoring your own feelings. This can be a balancing act of sorts because there may be times when you will feel uncomfortable—something difficult to avoid with growth and change. To make the changes you desire by using Bodycraft, it's important for you to work through those times of slight discomfort. However, be sensitive to the difference in a little discomfort versus your entire system shouting, "Whoa! Hold on! There is *no* way I am going to do this particular item."

The Structure

Bodycraft's structure is based on a series of five levels. Every level has four Bodycraft Tools, one for balancing each system: emotional, spiritual, mental and physical.

At the conclusion of a section, reasons are given for each tool and why it works. Some of these tools you will use for a lifetime, while others you may choose not to use at all. Still others may serve as a temporary bridge to get you where you want to go.

How to Use This Book

Read through the entire book; then return to work with each section. Live with each level's Bodycraft Tools for at least three weeks—that's the 21 days it takes to make a new habit—before going to the next level.

This approach provides a measure of comfort and avoids asking you to change so much or so quickly that it could become overwhelming. Also, this is a cumulative process, so you will continue using the tools from previous levels as you incorporate the new ones. If you need more time for any level, follow your instincts for what works for you.

At the end of each level is space for you to write any thoughts, ideas or feelings you have. There will also be the question: "What do I most need to know or do right now that is not here?" No one knows you better than you know yourself, and your inner knowing or intuition may surprise you.

Write it with your dominant hand. Then switch and write it with your non-dominant hand. Using each hand switches brain sides and can provide a different and insightful perspective.

Take the Time

Bodycraft doesn't make many demands, but it does require the commitment of a small portion of your time. If you are willing to dedicate a short period every day—some days as little as five minutes, some days up to an hour—it will work for you.

If that seems to be more time than you're comfortable giving, consider all the time you have dedicated to food (obsessing about it, preparing it, talking about it, hiding it); your weight (living every moment with the physical and emotional pain/discomfort, eternally seeking a book or weight-loss program that works, standing on the scale for the fourth time to get it to balance a half-pound lighter); and . . .well, need I go on?

When you think about it, a vast percentage of your life is consumed by food/weight/body issues, and it doesn't seem to make much difference whether it's about 10 pounds or 200 pounds. Isn't it worth taking a break from that for five to sixty minutes each day?

Additionally, be prepared to give Bodycraft and your body the time required for long-lasting change. In an instant society we have come to desire and expect instant results. However, abrupt changes can be a shocking jolt to your life, not to mention to your self-concept and identity. Like the birth of a baby occurring prematurely, rebirth before its time prevents the full development necessary to sustain it.

Gradual change gives you the opportunity to adapt to the different looks, feelings and directions of these changes, which can be considerable.

Expect (Unexpected) Changes

Creating new patterns in any area of your life may initially result in the appearance of the exact opposite of what you want. When that happens, it can be a sign that you're on the right track—even though it can be incredibly frustrating.

Our bodies and minds seem to maintain some inbred survival instinct to maintain the status quo (even a negative status quo), and the system works overtime to fight any threat of change. That is why at first you might feel you've taken one step back when you have been so diligently trying to go forward. Take heart, stick with it, and the desired change will occur.

As you continue with Bodycraft, there may be many positive changes that aren't immediately obvious. You may not even recognize such subtle changes until later as you look back.

You might also experience periods when there seems to be little or no change, followed by periods of rapid results. This is like to the stone mason who taps his or her hammer and chisel against the rock 99 times with no evidence of progress at all. On the hundredth tap, the rock easily splits into two pieces.

The keywords to your success in using Bodycraft are consistency and persistence. Whether you experience some quick and easy changes, or the more slowly evolving shifts, or some cord of both, the most important gift you can give yourself is to consistently pursue Bodycrafting that will serve you for a lifetime.

Relax

There are probably as many ways to relax as there are parts of the body. The simplest is the use of deep, rhythmic breathing. Here is one technique you can refer back to whenever relaxation is recommended.

Sit in a chair or on the floor with your spine straight. Imagine a cord dropping straight from the top center of your head through your tailbone down into the ground.

Close your eyes. Make your mind a white screen, clear of all thoughts and feelings. Take a deep, slow breath by inhaling slowly through your nose. Feel the incoming air inflating your abdomen slightly. At the completion of the inbreath, hold it briefly. Then slowly exhale until you have eliminated all of the stale air from your lungs.

At the completion of the outbreath, hold it briefly. Then, once again, inhale. Focus on the breath. Breathe slowly and deeply. Imagine with each in-breath that you are taking in love and light and the substance to create all you want in your life. On the outbreath, visualize releasing any tension, any negativity, anything no longer useful to you at this moment.

If distracting thoughts occur, calmly acknowledge and release them. Return your mind to being a blank screen at peace. Continue breathing.

Expect. . .

Expect only the very best of yourself and of Bodycraft. It is designed specifically to be pleasant, interesting and, above all, effective!

Level One

Weeks 1-3

Chapter Four

Bodycraft Tool #1: Self-Acceptance Now (Emotional)

Though we travel the world over to find the beautiful, we must carry it with us or we find it not.

-Ralph Waldo Emerson

It is a paradox that you must first wholly accept yourself before you can start making lasting change. If you are criticizing yourself and your body, you will create an internal rebellion that will never cooperate to achieve your desired body image. Any change made under those conditions will be temporary at best.

Love your body. Praise it. Revel in it. Regardless of what shape your body is, it deserves only your utmost love and respect. It has been with you every second of your life. It is always there for you. Think of each meaningful event in your life—a hug from a loved one, the smell of spring, the sound of soul-touching music, the vision of a violently colorful sunset. You can thank your body for every precious moment—every touch, smell, sound, sight, and taste—you have experienced in your life.

Even if you use loving and accepting yourself as a means in itself rather than as a vehicle for change, your life will be vastly enriched. The greatest gift you can have in life is being constantly delighted with yourself. We all deserve to live, love and be happy in all our many facets: with our great attitudes/bad moods, spiritual aspirations/agnostic doubts, perfectly toned forms/83% body fat, acne and warts/glowing skin.

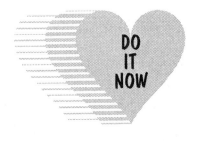

DO
IT
NOW

Right now go to a mirror and tell yourself aloud (or silently only if someone is around and you are embarrassed to be overheard) the following:

♡   I love my body because it lets me experience life.

♡   I am willing to love my body and myself without criticism.

♡ I am terrific, and I approve of myself exactly as I am right this minute.

♡ I am wonderful and lovable, and I love myself now.

♡ There are some changes I would like to make to enhance my life. If I make those changes, I will be perfect just as I am with them. If I don't make them, I will still be perfect just as I am. Changes are merely options that don't alter my basic perfection.

♡ I am exactly where I am supposed to be now, today, in this moment.

♡ I am a winner now and every day of my life!

Repeat these phrases with enthusiasm as you look at yourself in the mirror at least once every day, and preferably more often. Chant them. Sing them. Write them. Make them a part of you. Carry them in your heart and mind wherever you go.

There is a part of you that has waited a long time to hear this loving voice, and this exercise can hit some deep emotional chords. If contradictions or negativity come up, this exercise is just as valid since such feelings can show you areas needing your attention. If you cry, feel silly or even feel nothing, keep doing this process. Years of self-negation can take time to overcome, but this self-acceptance and self-love eventually sink in and come to stay.

Experiment using "you" or "I". As you look into the mirror and say, "You are wonderful and lovable, and I love you" or "I am wonderful and lovable, and I love myself", do you find one to be more effective or meaningful? Use what works best for you.

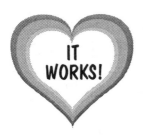

The reasons this emotional exercise is important in beginning your Bodycraft process:

1. It is only when you love and accept yourself as you are that you can make valid choices to create authentic and positive change.

2. After years of being told (and telling yourself) all the things wrong with you and your body, you may be talented at focusing on your perceived inadequacies. It is time to focus on the truth: you are lovable, and you are a winner *now*.

3. Feeling badly about yourself does nothing productive in your life. It isn't humility, but rather misdirected energy which projects a poor self-image to the world and holds you back. Alternatively, feeling good about yourself puts you on the high road to fulfilling all your potential.

4. Even if you don't initially feel in love with yourself and your body, the very act of doing this exercise is its own message of self-love.

5. You are in charge of your life. As you begin to genuinely love and respect yourself, your orientation changes. You are no longer running your life with the goal of seeking the approval of others, but rather living in ways that are best for you.

Bodycraft Tool #2: Blessing Your Food (Spiritual)

A single grateful thought towards heaven is the most perfect prayer.

-G. E. Lessing

This concept has many names and faces: focused human attention, prayer, blessing, healing words. It used to be considered exclusively religious. But recently there have been many impressive scientific investigations, research studies and analytical observations of these various concepts. They have been performed by such notables as Dr. William Tiller of Stanford University; Spindrift, Inc., a not-for-profit organization of Lansdale, Pennsylvania; and Larry Dossey, M.D., former chief of staff at Medical City Dallas Hospital, to name but a few.

There is a growing body of empirical evidence supporting what believers have known for centuries: prayer or blessing can have tangible effects in a material world. It's not just for church anymore.

Prayer/blessing is another Bodycraft tool which is easy, goes anywhere—and it's free! (Although as children we may have been coached to say our prayers and talk with God at night, the day rates are now just as inexpensive.)

Blessing takes practically no time—it can be as quick as your next thought. It has a positive effect on the blesser as well as on the blessed, and it raises your awareness even as it raises your food to a higher level.

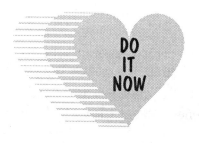

Bless every morsel you take into your body. Whether you're eating vegetables and organic brown rice or cola and chocolate cake, bless it before you consume it. Use a form of blessing that appeals to you personally. It doesn't have to be loud, wordy or pompous; but it can be. A momentary silent thought can be sufficient, or you may wish to use a special prayer.

My own method: I give a prayer of thanks for the food and drink, feeling gratitude to all those that took part in bringing it to me. I imagine it being filled with light and love and that it brings health, energy and vigor to my body. Sometimes I bless it silently, other times aloud.

Take that brief moment to bless your food and yourself, and over time, see the different it can make.

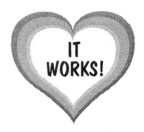

The reasons for blessing everything you take into you body:

1. The simple momentary act of blessing your food
   focuses your attention on it. This makes eating and
   drinking a conscious act, a choice, rather than a
   behavior without awareness—a small but important
   shift.

2. This allows you to start where you are now without
   changing your basic eating habits. You don't begin,
   as you may have on other programs, with the unpleas-
   ant and threatening commandment, "Thou shalt stop
   eating everything you like and commence eating food
   you detest."

3. You are raising the energy/vibration of whatever you
   are consuming, which will in turn ultimately raise
   yours. You will begin gravitating to food with a
   naturally higher vibration and nutritional value.

♥

Bodycraft Tool #3: Getting Your Mind Set (Mental)

Unless you know where you are going and why, you can't possibly get there.
                                                -*Warren Bennis*

When you take a trip, do you know *why* you are going? Even if you have left for a long journey with no planned destination, you're going for a reason. Maybe you love adventure. Perhaps you wish to experience family togetherness with your four children and two dogs in a compact car. Or possibly you want total freedom to see the country.

Indeed, the journey is the destination. But to take full advantage of the trip, it's best to have some idea of why you want to be on it in the first place.

Bodycraft is a major project and a great journey. It would be an excellent idea to know why you're doing this and exactly what you want to get out of it so you will have a personal blueprint to follow. That is the purpose of this exercise—it provides the structure for everything you want to accomplish with Bodycraft. At the same time, it has the flexibility to accommodate shifting needs and desires, and to change as you do.

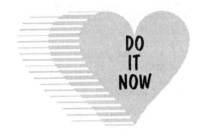

Think about and write down your Bodycraft goals and what benefits you expect from them. This includes how you want to think, feel, and behave differently. This tool helps you express these as tangible goals, while providing a mental "test drive" or "dress rehearsal" of your body as you want it to be.

Phrase these descriptions in positive terms and in the present tense. Instead of "I want to get rid of my fat thighs" or even "I will have the body I want", possible statements would include "My body *is* slender and well shaped. I now have strong, shapely thighs. I have great self-confidence. I walk standing tall and with a springy step."

Your mind is an efficient computer continually carrying out what you tell it with your words, feelings, and beliefs. That's why it is important to phrase in the present tense; otherwise the computer-mind may put your goal forever in the future. (Computers are so literal.)

Choose the phrases that fit your goals and desires. Be as detailed as possible, and as creative as you want to be.

Review these goals daily.

My goal(s) in crafting my body:

Why do I want this?

How my crafted body looks:

Having my body as I want it, here are some of the ways I think differently:

Having achieved the body I want, I also feel differently in many ways:

Some of the ways I behave differently with my crafted body:

Having this body which is perfect for me, I eat in ways that make me feel vibrant, nurtured and fulfilled. What and how do I eat food that I enjoy and feel good about to achieve that?

When any of your thoughts or goals change, write them down. You may notice some of your thinking/feeling/behavior goals are attainable now before you actually achieve any physical changes.

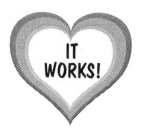

The reasons for this mental exercise of clearly stating goals in the present tense as positive affirmations:

1. You can only create something when you know what you want and why you want it.

2. The most effective way to get clear about what you want is to write it down.

3. Your physical being, thoughts, feelings and behavior (and self expectations of those) are intertwined. By changing any one of them, the others begin to follow.

Bodycraft Tool #4: Water (Physical)

Drink deeply of the water of Life, and you shall never thirst.

-Anonymous

Water is a miracle element that keeps your physical system clean and lubricated, washes out toxins, and fills you up but not out. That is only a small part of what water can do for you and your body.

Many experts agree that each day you need at least 1/2-ounce of water for each pound of your body weight. For example, if you weigh 160 pounds, you need a minimum of 80 ounces of water per day. That's if you are totally sedentary, live in a moderate climate and do not use caffeine, alcohol or other diuretics. If you are physically active or live in a hot climate, a daily intake of 2/3-ounce of water for every pound you weigh is recommended.

Those may sound like shocking amounts to anyone who currently drinks little or no water. Don't worry—you won't be asked to begin gulping down unmanageable amounts of the stuff. As with the entire Bodycraft process, this is geared to start from where you are without making overwhelming changes.

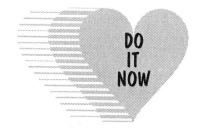

DO
IT
NOW

Start by drinking 8 ounces more water per day than you have been consuming. Each week add an additional 8 ounces per day until you are drinking the recommended daily amount of water. In other words, if you now drink no water, start with 8 ounces or one glass of water each day. After a week, increase your capacity to 16 ounces or two glasses of water daily. And so forth.

If you are a little fuzzy on measurements:

1 cup	=	8 ounces
1 pint	=	16 ounces
1 quart	=	32 ounces

If you are on the metric standard, you need about 35 milliliters water per kilogram of body weight or roughly 1.75 liters/50 kilograms. And if you are a person who refuses to measure anything, you can enjoy water in quantities measured by the liz standard of "a whole bunch" and "lots".

I strongly suggest drinking bottled water which is free of chlorine and chemicals and also (not surprisingly) tastes better. It can be purchased for very little from water vending machines (bring your own bottle) and very expensively if you prefer European vintage water.

My preference is distilled, but many people want the trace minerals available in spring water. If you can't get bottled water, tap water is still a viable alternative unless you are in an area with a water supply of questionable purity. (You can't get bottled water, and the tap water has all the tempting allure of a chemical spill? Where is this place, and how are you surviving? Can we airlift cases of Evian to you?)

According to Dr. Leroy R. Perry, Jr., Olympic Sports chiropractor and president of the International Sportsmedicine Institute in Los Angeles, "Water is vital for chemical reactions in digestion and metabolism and also lubricates our joints. By not drinking enough water, many people incur excess body fat, poor muscle tone, decreased digestive efficiency and organ function, increased toxicity in the body, joint and muscle soreness along with water retention."

Develop a taste for water if you haven't already. Be creative. Try it hot or iced. Flavor it with fresh-squeezed lemon. Enjoy the varied tastes of the many caffeine-free herb teas now available.

Another way to make drinking water more fun is by using colorful sports bottles. Check out biking bottles or the neon-colored quart bottles with the big plastic straws. They're inexpensive, unbreakable, and don't spill.

Partake of coffee, tea, milk or sodas as you wish—but they don't constitute water consumption. Each of these, while valuable to the survival of society as we know it, doesn't have the purely cleansing, hydrating properties of water.

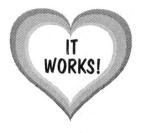 The reasons for adequate water consumption:

1. Weren't you paying attention to Dr. Perry ? He just gave you about a hundred good reasons (in the gray box). Did you notice the part about "incurring excess body fat" from lack of water?

2. Water purifies your system and moves out toxins and other waste products. For these reasons, it also supports a clearer skin tone.

3. It fills you up. Often when you feel hungry, it can be disguised thirst.

4. Elimination is improved.

5. Water may retard the aging process. A great deal of wrinkling and loss of skin elasticity have to do with the skin retaining inadequate moisture. If you're not drinking enough water to support the body's 65-75% water composition, something is going to dehydrate; and it will probably be the skin. That's only one small (vain) portion of aging. The rest of the body will no doubt also be maintained with greater quantity and quality of living if properly hydrated and lubricated.

P.S. On the other hand, getting carried away and drinking gallons of water daily isn't on the recommended list. Moderation in all things.

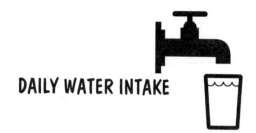

DAILY WATER INTAKE

Day 1_____   Day 8_____   Day 15_____

Day 2_____   Day 9_____   Day 16_____

Day 3_____   Day 10_____   Day 17_____

Day 4_____   Day 11_____   Day 18_____

Day 5_____   Day 12_____   Day 19_____

Day 6_____   Day 13_____   Day 20_____

Day 7_____   Day 14_____   Day 21_____

Your refrigerator is a good place to post this.

Level One Bodycraft Recap

After working with Level One Bodycraft Tools for at least three weeks, are you:

Emotional: ♡ Looking into the mirror to love and affirm your body and yourself at least once daily?

Spiritual: ♡ Blessing everything you put into your body?

Mental: ♡ Reviewing your described body image goals every day?

Physical: ♡ Gradually increasing your daily water intake up to 1/2-ounce per pound of body weight? (Divide your body weight by 2 and determine the minimum number of ounces of water you should ultimately be drinking on a daily basis.)

Before continuing to Level Two, examine your comfort level with each of these tools. If you are experiencing resistance or discomfort with any of them, you may want to focus additional time in that area, allowing it to become more workable for you. If the resistance or discomfort is extreme, let that part go for now.

When the Bodycraft Tools of Level One feel like a normal part of your life-style, it's time to move on to Level Two.

LEVEL ONE NOTES

Note here any thoughts, ideas or resistance you experience.

What is working for you?

What parts make you feel good?

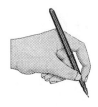 **. . . MORE LEVEL ONE NOTES**

Fully relax, then ask yourself: "What do I most need to know or do right now?" (Use first your dominant and then your non-dominant hand to write any answers that may come to you.)

AND JUST FOR YOU
. . . MORE NOTES

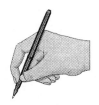

Level Two

Weeks 4-6

Chapter Five

Bodycraft Tool #5: Becoming
Your Future Now
(Emotional)

*Live now as you wish to be, for you are
now fully received into your future.*
                              -*Mohandas K. Gandhi*

If you ever played with a magnet under a paper
topped with iron filings, you saw the filings irresistibly
drawn to the position of the magnet. As the iron filings
clumped together on the paper, they took on the identical
shape—or made a "picture"—of the magnet underneath.

Think of your emotions as the magnet, your life the
paper, and circumstances/events the iron filings. The
emotional environment you create and that surrounds you
attracts the circumstances and events that form the
content—or picture—of your life.

Creating a permanent emotional environment that attracts and supports the kind of life you want—and applying this to your Bodycraft goals—also ensures changes which are long-lasting and stable. The following exercise shows you how to create that atmosphere.

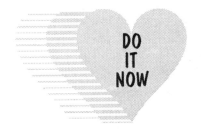

DO
IT
NOW

Select a place to be alone and quiet. When comfortable, close your eyes and relax. Imagine having the body image you described in the Bodycraft Tool #3 goal statements. What feelings would you experience? Would you feel happy, confident? What feelings would you have that you don't have now?

Make this experience and the feelings that go along with it as real and pleasurable as possible, and create the feeling that you are actually living it. Click. Make an internal emotional "photograph" of that feeling.

After you complete this experience, bring back the feelings and images of that emotional photograph; and as you go forward, *be* those feelings every moment of every day. Live with those sensations. If you lose the full impression, close your eyes and re-experience it.

> **Your feelings may shift or change from time to time, just as you and your goals do. Repeat this activity briefly once each day to keep the feelings fresh.**

This takes patience and persistence. At first your mind may scream, "Wait a minute, this isn't true!" These "I have already achieved" sensations initially can feel like wearing an ill-fitting suit; but if you keep using them, they will become perfectly tailored for you.

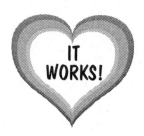

The reasons for building the feelings of having already achieved your desires:

1. Emotions are magnetic. You magnetize to you those things into which you put the most emotion.

2. Whatever you want, you must first become.

Bodycraft Tool #6: Reshaping Beliefs (Spiritual)

Man is what he believes.
-Anton Chekhov
. . .and so is woman.

You can hide what you think, but you can't hide what you believe. Beliefs are self-fulfilling prophecies, and beliefs you hold about your body are impossible to hide. (That doesn't stop us from trying to hide them, of course. Do you ever get disgusted with the whole camouflage routine and find that your closet full of slimming black and vertical stripes is becoming a huge bore? But I digress. . .)

You may be very aware of some of the beliefs you hold, and even verbalize them on a regular basis. Then there are those hidden beliefs that somehow crept in under the radar—you're living them without awareness that they exist.

This Bodycraft tool serves to take a clear look at your belief system. It allows you to decide which of those beliefs you want to emphasize and which you would like to replace. Then it shows you how to do so.

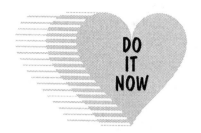

Spend five minutes quickly writing every thought that comes to you about your body and food.

Examples:
✦ All I have to do is look at food, and I gain weight.
✦ I hate my body.
✦ I have great legs.
✦ I feel fat.
✦ I can't live without chocolate sundaes.
✦ I have a lot of energy.

When you finish, read each statement and decide if you want to keep that belief. Then write it in present tense as a positive affirmation to fit the belief you want to have. Using the previous examples, the following would be possible affirmations:

♡ Food is a tool I use to nurture my healthy body.
♡ I appreciate my body which gives me life.
♡ I love how shapely and toned my legs are.
♡ I am sleek and fit.
♡ I sometimes choose to enjoy a chocolate sundae.
♡ I am full of energy.

Look at the statements on the first list. Imagine each belief you don't want to keep being erased and fading away until it is nothing.

Go to the positive affirmations on the second list. Say each aloud and make it part of you with all your senses—taste it, feel it, touch it, hear it, see it being you.

Include these affirmations with your goal statements. You may also want to record them on audiocassette—the sound of your own voice can have a powerful impact.

Periodically make a new list in order to bring out more beliefs to work with.

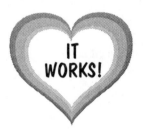

Why exploring your beliefs with affirmations is important:

1. First you have to find out what your deepest beliefs are. If you are mouthing cheery affirmations which are totally opposed to your underlying beliefs, you're driving with the brakes on.

2. When the belief is one you want to keep, it can be amplified and strengthened with affirmations.

3. If the belief is one you prefer not to have influencing your life, it should be acknowledged and removed. As long as the belief is there, it will be a roadblock to making change.

4. Once you eliminate the belief, you need to fill up that space with something else so the old belief won't slip right back in. The positive affirmation serves to do that.

5. It takes time to change a deeply ingrained belief, but by consistently removing the old belief and replacing it, the positive belief will take effect.

6. Your body and entire life are reflections of your belief system—so it becomes important to have beliefs that will build the kind of body and life you want.

Bodycraft Tool #7: Focused Daydreaming (Mental)

Only a dreamer can make a dream come true.
-Walt Disney

Do you know how to daydream? As children, we spontaneously daydreamed to create delightful friends and happy outcomes for our real and imagined adventures.

As adults, daydreaming still can be a sure bet for a good time, but the power it holds goes beyond even those positive results.

To understand the power of daydreaming, look at a few of history's great daydreamers and their legacies: Madame Curie, George Washington Carver, Joan of Arc, Albert Einstein, Leonardo da Vinci, Margaret Meade, Jesus Christ, Thomas Edison, Harriet Tubman, Walt Disney, Elizabeth Blackwell. We might conclude that a visionary is a daydreamer with a mission.

Who could doubt that Whoopi Goldberg as a welfare mother put abundant energy into daydreaming about becoming a famous, wealthy actress? And she followed a plan of action to make her daydreams a reality.

Daydreaming is relaxing and provides an outlet for the mind to see all possibilities, even in the so-called impossible.

There is one word that makes all the difference in whether daydreaming will be just a pleasant interlude, or a pleasant interlude which affords productive results. That word is "focus". Focused daydreaming means keeping to the subject of your goals and desires. It is still an unlimited arena. You can daydream about your highest dreams and desires to the most outrageous and in-depth lengths both possible and impossible. Focus also has to do with repeating these daydreams to your mind on a regular basis.

You could also call focused daydreaming "visualizing". They are essentially the same, except some people don't like the idea of visualization. "It's too hard." "I can't make mental pictures." "It's not fun." "It's too much work." (Although paradoxically, most of the people I know who claim to be incapable of visualizing their goals can clearly picture potential disasters in vivid detail. They refer to it as "worrying".)

Daydreaming is easy, everyone knows how to do it, and it's fun. Proceed now to (focused) Daydream Land.

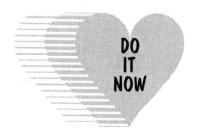

DO
IT
NOW

Relax. Think about the body you are crafting. (Refer to your goal statements and body description in Level One, Bodycraft Tool #3.)

Close your eyes, and for five minutes daydream as clearly as possible about how you want to look. (Imagine looking like your highest vision of yourself. To focus on looking like Heather Locklear if you resemble Bette Midler is counter-productive.)

If you need some "props", imagine looking at yourself in a mirror or seeing yourself in a movie. Daydream about how you look with that appearance.

Pay attention to the details. What are you doing, how are you acting, how are you standing? Do you walk or stride differently? Does your voice have a different tone? Do you act differently towards other people and expect to be treated differently? In your focused daydream adopt the entire persona of looking exactly the way you want to look.

Repeat this focused daydreaming at least once each day. Shortly after you wake up and right before you sleep are both excellent times.

When you're not involved in the process of focused daydreaming, *live* the dream. Take on the attributes of your daydreaming: the look, the stand, the voice, the behavior.

Have you noticed that fantastic-looking people often get to do more than those who are perhaps more ordinary in appearance? It's all in the attitude. Their looks merely give them the courage to believe they can; and they do. So get the attitude now, and the look will follow.

You can also incorporate the emotional activity of Bodycraft Tool #5 by feeling like you look that way now.

If your daydreams don't have pictures, fine. Use as many senses as you can to make it real, and the intent is enough.

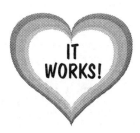

Why daydreaming is not only fun but also productive to Bodycrafting:

1. Daydreaming is a powerful tool for informing your mind of your goals in a relaxed and pleasant manner. As already discussed, your mind has a strong influence on all body functions.

2. When the mind has an attractive body image (or any other image), it will be true to the creation of that. Up until now, you may have experienced what happens by believing in an unattractive picture. Daydreaming teaches the mind to create the body you really want.

3. As with most learning processes, repetition is one of the best learning tools for the mind. It may take time and repetition for the mind to release the old picture

and replace it with the new one, so be patient and be persistent. For every bit of energy you put into this, you're replacing a small particle of the old picture with the new one. It's a cumulative process, and even if it feels as though nothing is happening at first, it is. Keep on keeping on, and the whole picture will form.

I have learned this at least by my experiment: that if one advances confidently in the direction of his dreams, and endeavors to live the life which he has imagined, he will meet with a success unexpected in common hours.

-Henry David Thoreau

Bodycraft Tool #8: Adopt a Food (Physical)

Discipline and focused awareness
contribute to the act of creation.
-John Poppy

If there were a pill that had all the benefits of satisfying hunger while promoting an attractive body and radiant appearance, the lines to the pharmacy would wrap around the block. There are such pills. They are rather large and some must be cut into smaller pieces. Opinions vary as to their pleasant taste. These "pills" are in your local grocery store, and they are the most inexpensive prescriptions you can buy.

They go by the collective name of produce. Fruits/ fruit juices. Vegetables/vegetable juices. Throw in some grains for good measure.

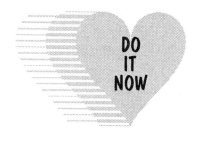

DO
IT
NOW

Here is your prescription: Eat them. Eat at least three servings of vegetables and three servings of fruit each day. Eat more if you like. If it's not too overwhelming for you, eat two or three servings of grains. The most important part, though, is the fruits and vegetables.

What is a "serving"? I personally prefer not dragging out measuring cups and scales. What do *you* think a serving is? Great! That's what it is for you. Make this easy on yourself, and recognize that these are merely guidelines that have worked for many people and that will probably work for you too.

Some individuals complain about not liking fruits or vegetables, especially vegetables. This can often be traced to childhood experiences with vegetables cooked to an unrecognizable pulp of indistinguishable color.

These upsets were compounded by parents who had the well-meaning nerve to say, "Eat them. They're good for you, whatever they are. I think they were peas before we boiled the life out of them."

You are a grown-up now, and it's time to put adolescent vegetable trauma behind you. Try different varieties of fruits and vegetables. Eat them raw. Sneak them into sandwiches. Sauté them. Make salads if you haven't come to despise the thought of a salad as "diet food".

If this is what it takes to start focusing on produce, deep fry it and dip it in cheese goo. Obviously, the closer to fresh and raw—unsweetened, unbuttered, unbattered, uncooked—the more nutritious most produce will be. But do what it takes to get started.

Did you know . . . ?
When fiber passes through your system, it carries with it about 10% of the fat present in the digestive tract—to be eliminated and never heard from again by your waist or thighs.

Plan ahead. If you don't stock fruits and vegetables in your refrigerator, you won't be eating them. Until it becomes ingrained, so to speak, think of it as a prescription that you need to buy ahead so you never run out.

Also plan when you intend to eat these foods, just like the now infamous prescription. It is so easy to be getting ready for bed and realize that you remembered to eat pizza and chocolate and a soda and a sandwich and a lot of other food; but, oh my, fruits and vegetables just completely flew out of your head. You need to have a solid intent backed by action to make this happen. Otherwise, it won't.

You know by now that Bodycraft is not about sacrifice and self-denial. It's not necessarily about taking the path of least resistance either, as in sinking into a big lethargic blob with no sense of values or direction.

This is about making choices that are best for the long run, while making you feel good in the present. I make these points so you won't go running into the sunset screaming, "It's just another diet book!" when the topic of food is approached. This is not about taking anything away. It is about adding foods that increase your well-being and enhance your appearance.

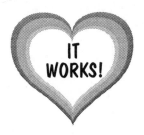

Why eat at least three servings each of fruits and vegetables (plus grains) each day?

1. First take note that nothing is being taken away from you. If you're still hanging on to your Milky Way, fine. (Remember to bless it.) I still enjoy chocolate and other "junk food". You may find that eating the "healthy" food displaces some of the junk simply because it can be satisfying both to taste and fullness.

2. Adequate nutrition is important to your health and good looks. It makes you feel fantastic, your skin glow, your hair shiny and alive, and life a lot easier to live than if you feel and look like hell. Fruits and vegetables can give you those benefits.

3. These foods are all high in fiber which means they are filling and satisfy hunger, as well as aiding regular elimination.

4. Fruits, vegetables and grains are obviously not the only important components of nutrition, but they are the most frequently neglected. I have found when I eat adequate amounts of these food groups, everything else falls into place nutrition-wise. The fruits, vegetables and grains are also the source of most vitamins and minerals. There are many excellent books available on food and nutrition if you are unaware of your basic nutritional needs and their sources.

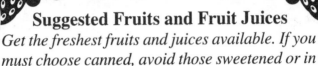

Suggested Fruits and Fruit Juices

Get the freshest fruits and juices available. If you must choose canned, avoid those sweetened or in syrup. However, those with sweeteners or syrup are preferable to none at all.

Apple/Apple Juice
Applesauce
Apricot/Apricot Nectar
Banana
Blackberries
Blueberries
Boysenberries
Cantaloupe
Casaba Melon
Cherries
Crabapples
Cranberries
Currants
Elderberries
Gooseberries
Grapefruit/Grapefruit Juice
Grapes
Guava
Honeydew Melon
Kumquat
Lemon

Lime
Loganberries
Loquats
Mango
Nectarine
Orange/Orange Juice
Papaya/Papaya Juice
Passion Fruit
Peach/Peach Nectar
Pear/Pear Juice
Persimmon
Pineapple/Pineapple Juice
Plantain
Plums
Pomegranate
Pricklypear
Quince
Raspberries
Strawberries
Tangelo
Tangerine
Watermelon

Suggested Vegetables and Vegetable Juices
Again, the fresher, the better.

Alfalfa Sprouts
Artichoke
Asparagus
Bamboo Shoots
Beets
Beet Greens
Broccoli
Cabbage
Carrots/Carrot Juice
Cauliflower
Celery
Chard
Collards
Cress
Cucumber
Dandelion Greens
Dock (Sorrel)
Eggplant
Endive
Green Beans
Kale
Kohlrabi
Leeks
Lettuce

Mushrooms
Mustard Greens
Okra
Onions
Parsnips
Peas
Peppers (Green/red/yellow)
Pumpkin
Radish
Rutabaga
Sauerkraut
Savoy
Spinach
Squash
Sweet Potato
Tomato/Tomato Juice
Turnips
Turnip Greens
Vegetable Juice
Water Chestnuts
Water Cress
Yams
Yellow Wax Beans

Grains
(Whole Grains Recommended)

These can be cooked individually or used as flours, cereals, breads, or pastas.

Barley
Bran
Buckwheat
Corn
Millet
Oats
Quinoa
Rice
Rye
Wheat

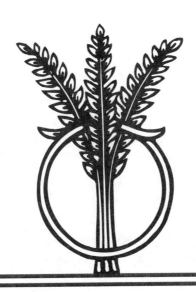

Level Two Bodycraft Recap

After working with Level Two Bodycraft Tools for at least three weeks, are you:

Emotional: ♡ Looking into the mirror to love and affirm your body and yourself at least once daily?

♡ Creating a permanent emotional environment that attracts and supports your Bodycraft goals?

Spiritual: ♡ Blessing everything you put into your body?

♡ Using affirmations to reshape beliefs?

Mental: ♡ Reviewing your described body image goals every day?

♡ Indulging yourself with the fun and productivity of focused daydreaming?

Physical: ♡ Gradually increasing your daily water intake up to 1/2-ounce per pound of body weight?

♡ Eating more fruits, vegetables and grains?

Before continuing to Level Three, examine your comfort level with each of these tools. If you're experiencing resistance or discomfort with any of them, you may want to focus additional time in that area, allowing it to become more workable for you. If the resistance or discomfort is extreme, let that part go for now.

When the Bodycraft Tools of Level Two feel like a normal part of your life-style, it's time to proceed to Level Three.

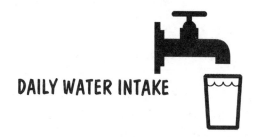

DAILY WATER INTAKE

Day 1_____   Day 8_____   Day 15_____

Day 2_____   Day 9_____   Day 16_____

Day 3_____   Day 10_____   Day 17_____

Day 4_____   Day 11_____   Day 18_____

Day 5_____   Day 12_____   Day 19_____

Day 6_____   Day 13_____   Day 20_____

Day 7_____   Day 14_____   Day 21_____

Your refrigerator is a good place to post this.

LEVEL TWO NOTES

Note here any thoughts, ideas or resistance you experience.

What is working for you?

What parts make you feel good?

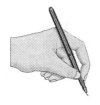

. . . MORE LEVEL TWO NOTES

Fully relax, then ask yourself: "What do I most need to know or do right now?" (Use first your dominant and then your non-dominant hand to write any answers that may come to you.)

AND JUST FOR YOU
... MORE NOTES

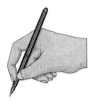

Level Three

Weeks 7-9

Chapter Six

Bodycraft Tool #9: Venting Your Rage to Live (Emotional)

The truth will set you free, but first it will piss you off.

-The Homemade Guru

In the book *Creative Aggression*, Dr. George R. Bach characterizes the newborn infant's first strident cry as the "rage to live" which starts the baby's breathing. *Rage to live.* What a magnificent description of the passion, glory and fire of being alive!

That is a stark contrast to the reality of how so many people exist. Those with impaired body images often conform to the expectations of others, shut down feelings for the sake of self-protection, and numb themselves in order to survive. That birthright of a "rage to live" eventually gets programmed out and deteriorates to a "lethargy to endure".

It is time to take back that birthright. It is time to be filled with passion for life and let every breath serve as a reminder of that first great howl when as an infant you demanded nothing less than to be fully alive.

Right. Easy to do is easy to say. But how?

By starting to fully feel again, you take back what is rightfully yours. What has been repressed and denied one emotion at a time, you take back one emotion at a time. First you recognize what emotions are there, and then you feel them. This section provides the tool to facilitate that process.

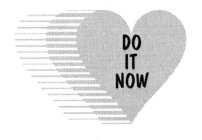
DO
IT
NOW

Start an "Emotions Journal". Write *something* in it every day about anything relating to your feelings/emotions. Write about how it feels to express (or not express) feeling glad, mad, sad or fearful. Write about how you stuffed the feeling or numbed yourself to it.

Here is just a sampling of what you might write about. Do you think it's okay to have feelings? Is it only okay to have certain feelings or no feelings? Do you deserve to have feelings (how many, which ones and how often)? Is it okay to express them? How is it okay (or not okay) to express them?

Write about feelings in your present as well as feelings in your past. Write about feelings you have about your body. Write about feelings you had about your body, eating issues, and the people and events relating to those issues from the time you were very young to the present.

After you journal about them, actually feel the feelings you have just written about.

These are ideas for getting started. They are your feelings, and it is your journal, so write and feel as little or as much as you want to. I encourage you to get started now and to do at least a small amount every day.

The Emotions Journal keeps your feelings flowing so that you experience them, get what information you need from them, and let them pass on through. The Journal also helps you flush out the areas where you are stuck so you can get unstuck and move on to grace.

Every feeling is fair game. If some feelings seem unethical or horrible (like the outrage that makes you wish your ex would get syphilis just before going bankrupt), remember that as you write them down they are safely contained on the paper and won't hurt anybody.

Getting in touch with anger can be incredibly therapeutic! In so-called polite society, anger has been regarded as an unacceptable emotion to feel, let alone to express. But that anger, even masked by a polite smile, goes somewhere. Maybe it gets pushed down and comes up at a later date in an uncontrollable fury. Possibly it turns inward and gives you migraine headaches or unending depression. Perhaps it just goes right to your hips. Is it worth the price to meet someone's outdated beliefs about "polite society" and "being nice"?

One can experience and express anger without being a raging maniac—in fact, without being impolite. A key element in successfully exercising any emotion, but particularly anger, is *appropriate* expression. Some misguided folks think being in touch with their feelings entitles them to be cruel, abusive, loud and obnoxious. WRONG. Appropriate expression allows all people concerned to maintain dignity and class.

Anger may need overt expression as well as journaling in order to be vented. Beating on a pillow and screaming can be effective in getting it out. My personal favorite is using a plastic bat to bash my mattress and yell. (I do this with my door closed and when no one else is in the house.)

One of my friends prefers putting ice cubes into a plastic bag and beating on the bag with a hammer. She gets her anger out and also has the added perk of crushed ice.

A revolutionary idea is to approach the person who is the recipient of this anger and calmly, firmly state, "I am angry at you for _____." (This is only if you feel safe both physically and emotionally—maybe even financially—to do so. There could be a vast difference in using this approach on a friend or a boss.)

There may be times either you feel you've opened a floodgate, or you feel nothing at all. Expect the pendulum to swing to both extremes. It may be scary (there's another feeling to write about), but it is also normal.

It might be helpful to enlist the aid of a therapist to guide you through any feelings you find challenging. This is a time to get extra support from people you trust and to double up on looking in your mirror to love and affirm yourself.

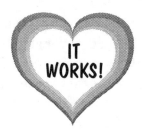

The reasons your Emotions Journal is vital to Bodycraft:

1. As stated at the beginning of this book, the body can be a red warning light for other systems. One of the biggest flashing red lights an impaired body image shows is that feelings have been stuffed, denied and in other ways not honored. Excess stored fat can also be viewed as excess stuffed emotions, or protective armoring.

2. Your Emotions Journal will begin making you aware of your true feelings even if you are stuffing, numbing or denying them. Awareness is the first step in honoring your right and need to feel, and appropriately express, your emotions.

3. It may not be fun when painful feelings surface, but you will be able to release them and quit carrying them with you everywhere—on your body and in your heart. The good news is that it also frees you to feel your joy.

4. Unfreezing emotions and getting them circulating releases great amounts of physical energy and also balances that energy. Getting the emotions unstuck can also get the body unstuck. And as you reclaim your physical and emotional energy, you will find yourself reclaiming your rage to live.

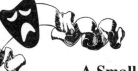 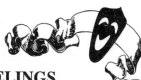

A Small Compendium of FEELINGS
(Not to be confused with the song often heard in bad piano bars)

Affection	Embarrassment	Love
Anger	Envy	Misery
Annoyance	Exasperation	Nervousness
Anxiety	Excitement	Panic
Apathy	Fear	Passion
Bitterness	Frustration	Peace
Bliss	Gaiety	Pity
Boredom	Gladness	Rage
Calmness	Guilt	Regret
Confidence	Happiness	Remorse
Confusion	Hatred	Repulsion
Contentment	Helplessness	Resentment
Curiosity	Hopefulness	Sadness
Delight	Hopelessness	Satisfaction
Depression	Hostility	Security
Despair	Humiliation	Serenity
Desperation	Indignation	Shame
Despondency	Indifference	Shock
Disappointment	Irritation	Surprise
Disgust	Jealousy	Terror
Dread	Joy	Trust
Eagerness	Liking	Worry
Ecstasy	Loneliness	Wrath

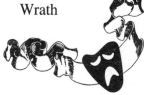

Bodycraft Tool #10: Meditation (Spiritual)

Meditation is not a means to an end. It is both the means and the end.
                                        -Jiddu Krishnamurti

When I first started meditating, I wasn't quite sure what to expect; but I did expect some moving experience that would change my life. Immediately. I thought I must be doing something wrong because nothing seemed to be happening.

As the years have passed, I have been able to see the subtle yet dramatic impact of meditation. I have a greater clarity of thinking, more inner peace and calmness, and a higher sense of purpose. I feel closer to a Higher Power and a sense of order in the universe. Meditation has many benefits, but it has not made me a saint. Among other unsaintly traits, I still fidget and snarl in rush hour traffic—but not quite as much.

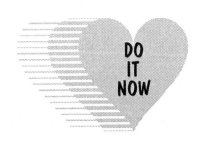

DO IT NOW

Try meditation for yourself. There is a vast array of methods for meditating, and there are many books available on the subject. This is another of those processes that is

almost impossible to do wrong as long as you are extend-
ing the effort to do it at all. If you have no previous
meditation experience, a few simple techniques follow.

♡ *Find a quiet place free of distractions. Sit comfortably with your spine straight. Close your eyes, and
still the mind. Relax and begin breathing slowly and
deeply. Practicing this for 5 to 30 minutes each day
is a simple and effective form of meditation.*

The following are other methods you may wish to use:
(Don't suffer a marathon meditation by trying to do them
all at once.)

♡ *Imagine your mind becoming a blank screen, and
focus on maintaining that state. As thoughts come to
your mind, don't become critical of the thoughts or
of yourself for having them. Simply bless and release
them. Then return to the blank screen.*

♡ *Light a candle (in a safe place away from any
flammable materials, please!) and focus on the
flame. Maintain thoughts only of the candle flame.
As other thoughts intrude, bless them and let them
go. Return your one-point focus to the flame.*

♡ *Visualize yourself walking down a beautiful flight of
stairs with ten steps. Walk down each one. 10 - 9 - 8
- 7 - 6 - 5 - 4 - 3 - 2 - 1. See how beautiful you are
surrounded by golden light. At the bottom of the*

steps, you come to a hallway filled with the same golden light. Begin walking down the hallway.

The light changes to a clear red. Walk through the red light, and feel it warming you; breathe it in, let it surround you. The light changes to orange. Walk through the orange light. Feel it, breathe it in, taste it. Do this in turn with yellow, green, blue, indigo, purple and finally white light. Experience each one with as many senses as you can.

At the end of the hall, there is another flight of 10 stairs you may ascend. 1 - 2 - 3 - 4 - 5 - 6 - 7 - 8 - 9 - 10. Whenever you are ready, open your eyes. (See Appendix B.)

♡ *Focus on your breathing. "See" the breath coming in and going out. Imagine love and light and good coming in with each inhalation. As you exhale, imagine releasing everything you no longer need or want in your life.*

♡ *Focus on your perception of God, Higher Power, Higher Self or love. Feel yourself surrounded and filled with perfect love and peace.*

♡ *Imagine being in the most beautiful room you have ever seen. It is your special room, and it is yours to use anytime you want to meditate or feel peaceful. Maybe you prefer an outdoor setting. Whatever you choose, make it personally significant and completely your own.*

♡ *If the empty mind or "blank screen" is challenging, start by focusing on the good things in your life one at a time. If you feel stuck about where to start, think about simple things you take for granted. Reflect on having breath and life in your body, friends you like, family you love, a place to live, having enough to eat, your favorite music, a beloved pet. This is otherwise known as "counting your blessings". When you really stick with this, you can change even a lousy, rotten mood into a deep sense of appreciation for your life.*

If you are human and living on Planet Earth, it is likely that during the first many attempts to meditate your mind will wander around like some kid lost in a shopping mall. The sooner you can let it be okay that you may be slightly unfocused, the easier it will be to refocus. This is a natural part of the process.

You may want to record your special meditation on audiocassette. There are also many professionally-performed guided meditations available on tape at bookstores and some music stores.

Perhaps there are other types of meditation more suited to you. The late Joseph Campbell said that his personal form of meditation was underlining favorite passages in books.

Meditation is a special time just for yourself, to feel happy and at peace. If you are achieving that, you are meditating.

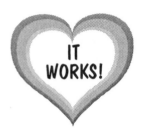 Why meditation is important to your Bodycraft process:

1. Meditation is a choice tool for balancing all of the systems—spiritual, mental, emotional and physical.

2. Meditation puts life into perspective. It gives a time and method for shrinking mountains to a manageable size.

3. This is a special time and experience you do just for yourself. It is a time to fully "own" yourself, your

body, your time and to realize your life and body are completely yours to direct.

4. Meditation puts you fully in touch with yourself and the infinite. It presents a time to love and appreciate yourself and your body just as you are right now. It is a gift of the miracle of you.

Bodycraft Tool #11: Treasure Mapping (Mental)

*Castles in the air are necessary before we
can have castles on the ground.*
-Ralph Waldo Trine

So far, most of your work at the mental level has been to reprogram the amazingly efficient computer of your mind. Level One involved using words to direct it, and Level Two employed internal pictures through focused daydreaming. With a process called "treasure mapping" you will now be using external pictures to represent your goals.

There are infinite ways this can be done, so consider the following as guidelines to "run and play" in ways that feel good and are fun for you.

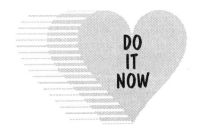

Create a picture of how you will look when you have crafted your body image as you want it. You can draw the pictures, cut them out of magazines or take them from any source you find appealing. The treasure map will be most effective if the pictures resemble your features as closely as possible.

You can make your treasure map large or small. Using a size which fits into a three-ring binder allows you to create an entire collection. Construction paper or poster board make good backgrounds.

When you have the picture(s) on your treasure map, write affirmations on or around them. The positive goal statements you made in Bodycraft Tool #3 and the affirmations of Bodycraft Tool #10 would be ideal to use. Integrating these different processes is not only more efficient and requires less time, but also intensifies the results as they work together. You may also consider incorporating some symbol of your Higher Power into your treasure map.

Look at the treasure map at least once daily and repeat the affirmations. Think about it periodically throughout the day. This can also be complementary to use with your focused daydreaming.

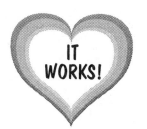

The reasons creating a treasure map can be instrumental in crafting your body:

1. It creates a clear, tangible picture of what your goal is and gives it a greater sense of reality.

2. Putting the energy into creating this on paper (or the medium of your choice) gives you the symbolic message that this is a goal you are committed to creating on a physical, three-dimensional level as well.

3. It acts as a physical blueprint for your ultimate outcome. From this blueprint, your subconscious and conscious minds begin generating the energy to physically create the results.

Bodycraft Tool #12: The Breath of Life (Physical)

Keep breathing.
-Sophie Tucker regarding her secret to a long life

What could be more basic than breathing? It is more important and immediate to your survival than any other resource. You can live without food for over a month, and even the necessary magic of water can be sacrificed for as long as four days. Your system would stop functioning, however, if you were deprived of breath for longer than four minutes.

The breath maintains the perfect chemical balance of oxygen and carbon dioxide in your system. It sends life-giving oxygen to your blood, gives energy, clarity and cleansing to every cell of your body. Breath is the basic building block of energy and is considered an automatic or autonomic response. That doesn't imply you have no control of this process. Quite the contrary, you have extraordinary freedom in modifying and enhancing your breathing.

Unfortunately influenced by tension, poor posture and inattention, most people have gone the wrong way by becoming shallow breathers, frequently using less than one-fifth of their lung capacity.

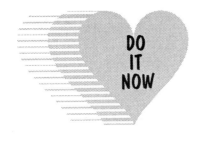

It is time to focus attention on what is literally the breath of life and redirect the trend of underusing it. A simple beginning breathing exercise follows:

Lie flat on your back. Relax. Place one palm on your abdomen. Exhale slowly, moving every last bit of stale air out of your lungs, pushing (but not straining) with your diaphragm and abdominal muscles. (Exhaling is actually more important than inhaling. Once the old stale air is completely eliminated, fresh air will rush in to fill the vacuum.)

Inhale, filling the lower part of your lungs, then the middle, then the top. Think of it like filling a cup from the bottom up. When you are doing this properly, you should feel your abdomen rising slightly under your palm. Your abdomen is the only part of your body noticeably moving—the head, shoulders and chest should remain still.

Repeat this exhale/inhale cycle slowly and fully for a few minutes.

Once you become accustomed to this deep breathing pattern, you can do it anywhere: in traffic, while walking, at the office. The possibilities are endless. You have to breathe, so you may as well do it to your greatest advantage.

If you wish to learn and experience more about breathing, take some yoga classes. Hatha yoga is based on the integration of breath with body movement. It's gentle enough for almost anyone to do, and it is highly recommended for even those who are physically challenged.

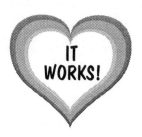

Consistently breathing fully and deeply is important because:

1. It energizes the system, improving circulation, complexion, digestion and energy levels.

2. Full breathing increases oxygen to all parts of the body and eliminates those ugly toxins. Oxygen intake is important to anyone's general health, but if you are reducing stored fat, it is of particular importance. Burning fat requires the presence of adequate oxygen, similar to the requirements for starting a

fire. As part of that fat-burning process, oxygen (like water) is also needed to remove the resulting waste products from your body.

Note: Be sure you have adequate iron in your diet to form the red blood cells that carry the oxygen.

3. Proper breathing puts you in touch with the most basic core of your existence and thus helps you connect with your emotions. It provides a centering, stabilizing force and can have a calming effect if some emotions feel uncomfortable or overwhelming.

Level Three Bodycraft Recap

After working with Level Three Bodycraft Tools for at least three weeks, are you:

Emotional: ♡ Looking into the mirror to love and affirm your body and yourself at least once daily?

♡ Creating a permanent emotional environment that attracts and supports your Bodycraft goals?

♡ Using your Emotions Journal daily and reclaiming the Rage to Live?

Spiritual: ♡ Blessing everything you put into your body?

♡ Using affirmations to reshape beliefs?

♡ Finding the perspective of meditation?

Mental: ♡ Reviewing your described body image goals every day?

♡ Indulging yourself with the fun and productivity of focused daydreaming?

♡ Treasure mapping?

Physical: ♡ Gradually increasing your daily water intake up to 1/2-ounce per pound of body weight?

♡ Eating more fruits, vegetables and grains?

♡ Breathing fully?

Before continuing to Level Four, examine your comfort level with each of these tools. If you're experiencing resistance or discomfort with any of them, you may want to focus additional time in that area, allowing it to become more workable for you. If the resistance or discomfort is extreme, let that part go for now.

When the Bodycraft Tools of Level Three feel like a normal part of your life-style, it's time to go to Level Four.

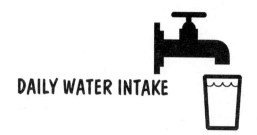

DAILY WATER INTAKE

Day 1_____   Day 8_____   Day 15_____

Day 2_____   Day 9_____   Day 16_____

Day 3_____   Day 10_____   Day 17_____

Day 4_____   Day 11_____   Day 18_____

Day 5_____   Day 12_____   Day 19_____

Day 6_____   Day 13_____   Day 20_____

Day 7_____   Day 14_____   Day 21_____

Your refrigerator is a good place to post this.

LEVEL THREE NOTES

Note here any thoughts, ideas or resistance you experience.

What is working for you?

What parts make you feel good?

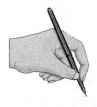

. . . MORE LEVEL THREE NOTES

Fully relax, then ask yourself: "What do I most need to know or do right now?" (Use first your dominant and then your non-dominant hand to write any answers that may come to you.)

AND JUST FOR YOU
...MORE NOTES

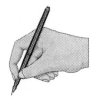

Level Four

Weeks 10-12

Chapter Seven

Bodycraft Tool #13: The Power of Your Hidden Emotions (Emotional)

As you follow the thread of your feelings, you will find a little more of yourself every day.

Current brain/body studies indicate that everything an individual has ever experienced mentally, physically and emotionally is forever programmed into his/her brain. Furthermore, through the nervous system, these messages become part of the body at a cellular level.

Thus each thought, experience and feeling you have ever encountered is indelibly etched on every cell of your body. This should give you a clue that the body has some powerful information to share.

Although we are aware of much of this information, some of it is lurking below the conscious level. That's the part that can disable all our good intentions.

If we operated on a purely conscious level, we would always do only those things in our best interests. In such a conscious world there would be no nail biters nor addicts. Obviously, there is a lot going on beneath our awareness that can sabotage our most passionate (conscious) desires and highest goals.

This tool is designed to tap into emotions stored in your body and discover why they are undermining your desired body image—and maybe other goals as well. You can bring those hidden dynamics to light and harness their power to work for rather than against you.

First recognize that all of your behavior is based on positive intent. It may be twisted, and it may be working against you; but at some point it started as a way to benefit you. An example of this from my life:

> *As a small child my parents insisted I clean my plate under the threat of spankings. It made all kinds of sense at the time to ignore the protests of my full stomach and protect myself by eating everything on the plate. Also, displaying a big appetite and eating received a great deal of positive attention in our family.*

My unconscious belief that overeating was a way of both protecting myself and getting positive strokes continued long past its effectiveness. Think of how powerful that ingrained emotion must have been to later override my obsession to have a slender body, my conscious belief that overeating was undesirable, and my fears of societal disapproval. Imagine what can be accomplished when the force of such a powerful belief is used as an ally.

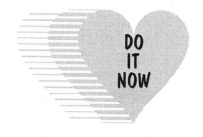

This process combines two methods of going beyond the conscious: use of the non-dominant hand and drawing pictures. This isn't designed to produce work suitable for gallery display. It's not even for public viewing unless you choose to share it with someone who fully supports you. This is a tool to assist you in reaching your goals.

Allow whatever comes out to be exactly what it is: an expression that tells you more about yourself.

Using the non-dominant hand will initially be slow, illegible and irritating. Be patient, and just let it happen. This is a highly effective way to reach normally inaccessible information about yourself.

I recommend using colored markers (the Mr. Sketch felt-tipped markers are my favorite), but crayons, colored pencils, pastels, paint or any medium will work as long as you can make pictures with it. Paper is a nice touch too. (If you want to try other backgrounds and don't mind what the neighbors say about your unusual wall murals, there really is no limit to what you might try.)

♡ *Using your non-dominant hand, draw a picture of how you perceive your body. Draw the front. Draw the back.*

♡ *Close your eyes and relax. Slowly move the focus of your attention throughout your body. Take a careful physical and emotional inventory of each area. When you are finished, open your eyes and stretch.*

Using either hand you choose, write any impressions or feelings you experienced in any part(s) of your body.

♡ *With your dominant hand, write questions to different parts of the body. Write the answers with your non-dominant hand.*

The following is an excerpt from my impressions of a "body inventory" I did some years ago:

"I see a really well-shaped body with a large stomach. The face is both happy/sad = perplexed. The stomach feels a need to be bigger because this is the Center for Creativity. It feels a need to shout, 'Hey! Look at me!' in some way for recognition and validation of that creativity. It usually feels ignored

& the stepchild of the body & the energy. It just wants some attention. It represents the child inside and the child's creativity but also that of the adult. PAY ATTENTION TO THE CHILD! PAY ATTENTION TO THE CREATIVITY. NURTURE BOTH & GIVE THEM OUTLETS."

My stomach was always the bane of my appearance, and I obsessed over it for years. Even the rare times when a diet succeeded and I became slender, regardless of how many sit-ups and abdominal crunches I did, that pot belly would never completely go away.

This exercise helped me hear the message it had been trying to deliver. With some resistance, I started allowing myself creative expression through journaling, drawing pictures (which I struggled not to judge), writing and any means that I could consider a way of expressing who I am and what I am about.

I started honoring and loving my stomach as a blessed gift rather than as a hated enemy and gave thanks for this creative center which had given me the great gift of creating a new life. Due to my long-standing habit of self-criticism, I did not experience an immediate change of attitude.

This journey has been a small miracle. I have found great joy in my creativity and an abundance of self-love through these processes. I have even discovered some artistic talent under the layers of denial. And, yes, my stomach I learned to love as it was, has receded to a slight roundness.

The following is an example of left/right hand dialogue with two body areas. Questions reflect dominant hand use, answers non-dominant:

Q: *What is causing the forehead to be tight & worried?*

A: *It thinks too much. Its job is to figure out what can go wrong. Crappy job. Long hours. Lousy pay.*

Q: *Why are the cheeks & mouth & chest so happy?*

A: *They LOVE being happy. That's their job. But sometimes it's not ok to be too happy where people notice. Like laughing loud & singing & jumping around. So they tone it down. Like when the forehead says, "Y'all be quiet so I can hear myself worry. This is serious & more important than being silly." The forehead is a dumbjerk.*

Q: *Let's talk to the forehead. How do you feel about your job & how the "happy" parts view you?*

A: *I try to keep order & prevent anything bad from happening. It keeps us all out of trouble. I would like to be happy but I don't have time. Plus the others are too loud & silly. I worry about what people think.*

Q: *It seems your job then is to keep unhappy things from happening.*

A: *Well, yes.*

Q: *So in a sense you're trying to keep things happy.*

A: *Well, I guess so.*

Q: *But you're unhappy, which makes your entire job a Catch-22. Have you thought of maintaining a quiet happiness (rather than the boisterousness you dislike) or at least peacefulness while you do your job? And instead of conjuring up possible horrors, just stay alert for problems. . .seeking positive possibilities. . .because what you think about is usually what happens.*

A: *I'll try it. Please help me learn to laugh.*

Approach this process with no preconceived ideas of outcome. Let it flow with misspelled words, bad grammar, corny lines or even complete silliness.

When you identify a concept working against you, dialogue with that part to find out what its positive intent is. Then discover how you can use that concept as a win/win to achieve the original positive intent. At the same time it can help you reach your current (conscious) goals it may previously have been working against.

———————

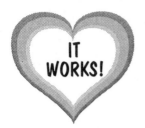

The reasons tapping body emotions with drawing and non-dominant hand dialogue works:

1. This makes it possible to uncover unconscious intents which may be sabotaging your goals. It works to get that under-the-surface "gunk" unstuck, like an emotional Roto-Rooter.

2. It helps find ways to use those powerful intents (previously working against you) to positively support what you want to create in your life.

3. It can bring underlying needs, wants and even abilities to the light of conscious understanding.

Bodycraft Tool #14: OA or Other Support Group (Spiritual)

I get by with a little help from my friends.
-*John Lennon & Paul McCartney*

One of the greatest burdens of an impaired body image is the sense of isolation that goes with it. Good support groups provide relief for leaving the burden of aloneness at the door and being surrounded by loving, compassionate people who have experiences similar to your own.

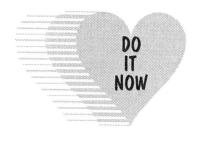

One way to end the lonely battle is to attend Overeaters Anonymous (OA) meetings or any other appropriate support group for body issues. (See Appendix A.) OA is a Twelve Step program and one of the few places to recognize the entire human-ness of the person with an eating disorder.

With OA, you will not be charged a fee. You will not be handed a diet program. You will not be told you need more willpower or more "won't power". (It *will* be suggested you try a Higher Power.)

You won't have to identify yourself or give any information other than what you volunteer, and you won't be required to attend a certain number of meetings.

You *will* be among people who share the same problems you do with body, weight and food issues. These people also share many of the same strengths you have: the recognition that they deserve to treat themselves and be treated by others with dignity; courage to face their innermost selves and make changes from the inside out; determination to heal their wounds no matter how long it takes or what anyone else's opinion about it may be; the knowledge that they are precious, valuable human beings who deserve rich, happy lives.

OA is a safe place to get support in healing old wounds.

You can find OA in the telephone directory. Each meeting has its own personality, so if you don't like one, try different meetings until you find one that fits you.

Or start your own OA group. You can get information from:

Overeaters Anonymous
World Service Office
P. O. Box 92870
Los Angeles, California 90009
(310) 618-8835

[At the time of this printing, OA's World Service Office has plans to move to Albuquerque, New Mexico, but has not yet established either a new telephone number or address. If you are unable to reach them with the above information, try Albuquerque directory assistance at (505) 555-1212.]

Phone lists are available at OA meetings which provide the names and numbers of members who are open to sharing support. This phone list is a source for enlisting nurturing, sharing and help from others. If you feel you are imposing to call someone, remember the reason the list exists is so you *can* call.

Common courtesy and common sense should, of course, prevail. When you call, ask if it's a good time (3:00 a.m. is seldom a good time for anyone). If that person cannot talk, and assuming it is a reasonable hour, call someone else on the list. Honor the person's time by being brief. When I receive such a call, I'm uplifted by the trust it shows; and I always learn and grow from what that person shares. It's a two-way street—so you're actually supporting someone else's growth, as well as your own.

I recommend OA whether you are 500 pounds overweight or 50 pounds underweight. As paradoxical as that may sound for an "overeaters" program, any body image problem associated with food and/or weight obsession has similar origins.

If OA is not for you, look for other support groups that you do feel comfortable with. Watch bulletin boards and flyers in the places you frequent, or look in bookstores and natural food stores for such information. And if that special group doesn't materialize, start your own Bodycrafters support group.

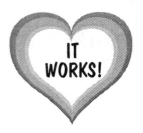

The reason it is worth your time to find OA meetings or another appropriate support group to attend:

1. A good support group for food/body issues breaks the sense of isolation you may have experienced. You learn that you are not alone, and that you *do* belong.

2. OA is a spiritual program (not religious, but spiritual), and there is great power and release in recognizing you do not have to do it on your own. To trust a Higher Power, however you perceive it, is self-actualizing and facilitates changes you wish to make.

3. This is a place to feel safe and to dump any shame or fears you may have around your issues. Nothing is judged negatively in these meetings. And hearing other people's stories, even if you choose not to share, is healing.

4. You're liberated to have the support without having to swallow any "shoulds" regarding what you should eat, how you should act or how much you should weigh. You can receive support in determining some of your own guidelines, if you wish.

Bodycraft Tool #15: Reclaiming Your Mind-Body Voice (Mental)

We ate when we were not hungry and drank without the provocation of thirst.

-Jonathan Swift

One of our greatest challenges is reconciling what food our bodies really want with what food our mouths are clamoring for. Sometimes there is an enormous chasm between the two demands.

Bodycraft Tool #15 is a process I call "using the mind-body voice" and, as the term implies, has overlapping mental and physical boundaries. It employs a mental process to achieve body consciousness.

This "mind-body voice" concept came about as a result of often feeling like I wanted something to eat, but nothing seemed quite right. I would mentally go over every conceivable food I thought I wanted, and nothing struck a chord as being the perfect piece (peace?) of food.

Sometimes I would taste test to be sure, and even ice cream or my ever-beloved peanut butter (yup, with a spoon right out of the jar) would leave me dissatisfied. How incredibly frustrating!

There were a few clearheaded occasions when on some level I was asking myself, "Okay, so what do you really want?" And the answer would come back, "water" or "nothing". Or I would get a clue that maybe since nothing sounded good, nothing was what would be good. Those times when I recognized and (this is the tough part) accepted it, I felt entirely satisfied. I may have initially felt somewhat frustrated because I was not filling the hole in my soul with food; but there was something about that recognition and doing what was my genuine desire that created its own sense of fulfillment.

There were also times I would get mental pictures of some type of food my body wanted. Whenever I indulged such a "nudge", it tasted right, was completely satisfying, and I felt gratified that I was doing something good for myself.

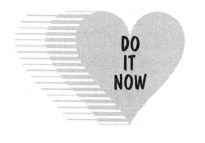

DO IT NOW

Now is the time to pay attention to what your body has to say. This will be an individual matter of paying attention to yourself and your inner messages. Some tips for getting started:

♡ *Mentally ask your body, "What do you want right now?" Be centered, focused and receptive to an answer that may come in words, pictures or feelings. It may even be something other than food, such as rest or sleep, companionship, exercise or a change of view.*

♡ *When you have a choice of foods, first mentally picture each food and your response to it. Mentally taste the food. Imagine what your body thinks about receiving any of these foods.*

♡ *Think of this food becoming a part of your body— tomorrow's new cells, toned muscles and glowing skin.*

♡ *Learn to assess your hunger level. Imagine a measure similar to your car's fuel gauge or a scale of 1 to 10 to estimate how full your stomach is. Empty or a 1 would be gnawing, almost painful hunger. Half-full or a 5 would be comfortably full. If you are at Full or a 10, you are painfully full, and your consuming desire is for a larger waistband.*

Experiment. Notice how you feel at each level. Observe your hunger level when you start eating. Do you feel best when you begin at a 7 or three-quarters of a tank? Or is it actually more pleasant to wait until you are at 2 or 3 and closer to Empty? Where is your hunger level as you eat, and then when you finish eating? If you feel great after a meal, observe where that level is. If you are at a 10 (or at a 1

because you insist on abusing yourself with some
starvation plan) and feel wretched, simply observe
the level and feelings without judgment.

This is information for you to decide how you
want to eat and what makes you feel best. Most people
are shocked to discover that eating is more pleasurable
when they are slightly hungry, and that hunger does not
bring on sudden death.

You may find this to be another process that takes
some time and observation to master. As with most
Bodycraft execises, it requires persistence—not perfection. Initially, you may find checking in with your body
is sporadic at best. Then even as you become more
consistent about checking it out, what the mouth wants
may win out if there is a conflict. Or you may ask what
your body wants and be unable to distinguish the answer.

As you persist in paying attention, you will get
clearer messages. As you eat what feels right, you'll
discover the food is perfect for what you really want.
And even the mouth (which may initially disagree) will
ultimately be happy. This track record of satisfying the
body, soul, and even the mouth, will encourage you to
listen and follow through with the message.

Be as honest with yourself as possible as to what
messages are coming from where.

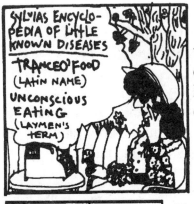

SYLVIA'S ENCYCLO-
PEDIA OF LITTLE
KNOWN DISEASES

TRANCEO'FOOD
(LATIN NAME)
UNCONSCIOUS
EATING
(LAYMEN'S
TERM)

A SUFFERER SPEAKS:

"OFTEN THE FIRST THING I NOTICE IS THAT MY JAWS ARE MOVING. THEN I LOOK DOWN AT MY HAND AND THERE'S A PIECE OF COFFEE CAKE IN IT."

ANOTHER SUFFERER SPEAKS

"I WAS DRIVING 85 MILES PER HOUR ON THE FREEWAY, WHEN I NOTICED I WAS EATING. I WAS COMPLETELY BAFFLED. THEN I SAW THAT MY GLOVE COMPARTMENT WAS STUFFED WITH CHILI DOGS.

Suppose the body wants broccoli, and the mouth wants chocolate; and you decide on the chocolate. Recognize that you made a choice you are entitled to make without judging that it was good or bad. (This is a nice way of saying not to torture yourself with guilt). Observe how you feel about your choice. That honesty will avoid distortion of the messages, and keep you attuned to yourself.

This is like any other tool: it is there to assist you, but you may not always choose to apply it. Deciding not to use it is no reason to bend the tool and make it unusable for future service.

Your body never lies, but it is up to you to hear its message. If the body's voice has long been silenced, ignored, and shamed, it may no longer speak quite as audibly as it once did. As you give it the respect of listening to and following its wisdom, it will speak with ever greater clarity.

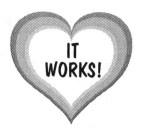

Why reclaiming your body-mind voice is important:

1. It honors and respects the body, and the body responds positively to that treatment just as you do to people who treat you with respect and listen to you.

2. It attunes you to your highest level of needs and wants. You will have a greater chance of achieving fulfillment if you know what needs fulfilling. (I.e., your food will taste better, and you will eat what you really

want. This definitely beats eating three loaves of fat-free oat bran bread then wondering why you don't feel satisfied.)

3. Listening to your body and its desires gives you focus on what you are consuming. Even if you choose to eat something other than what your body wants/needs, it is a conscious choice rather than unconscious response.

Bodycraft Tool #16: Exercise (Physical)

Thomas Jefferson said that not less than two hours a day should be devoted to exercise. If the man who wrote the Declaration of Independence, was Secretary of State, and twice President, could give it two hours, [we] can give it ten or fifteen minutes.

-John F. Kennedy

If you have never considered the remote possibility that the words "fun" and "feel good" could logically appear in the same sentence as "exercise", I beg your indulgence in taking a fresh look at the whole process.

I, too, used to consider exercise with as much appreciation as major surgery or being in a five-hour holding pattern over Chicago. Doing stupid calisthenics, huffing, puffing, feeling klutzy and inept—isn't it amazing I could resist such an attractive picture?

My eternal quest for weight control and a slender body finally drove me to the (one of many) last-ditch efforts of exploring exercise. I read a book which glamorized the wonders of running, and with a non-existent fitness level, I started running a couple miles a day. It was a horrible ordeal, and I quit—fortunately, before I did any serious damage to myself.

Two years and several extra pounds later, desperation drove me to try again. This time a friend who coached track advised me to do it gradually and recommended a simple, step-by-step program. His final dictate was a blessing that should be bestowed upon anyone engaged in any endeavor, but particularly an exercise program: "When you get tired, or if you feel any pain, stop immediately."

I *slowly* increased my stamina, endurance and distance. There were times when I worked through boredom or slight discomfort; but I was never in pain, and I never felt awful. In fact, I almost immediately started feeling better.

That was 11 years ago. I now run a few miles each week or occasionally bike or do aerobics for a change of pace. I do some easy weight training that takes less than 15 minutes each day. I exercise consistently, but I don't knock myself out.

At one point in my exercise evolution, I went through a phase of exercise mania that, as most obsessions do, made me sick and miserable and not much more fit. (That seems typical for me: I often have to experience both extremes of the spectrum before I find a workable place somewhere in the middle.)

The following is the simple exercise/fitness philosophy I shaped from these experiences:

♡ *A basic level of fitness is essential.*
♡ *It better be fun.*
♡ *It can't take up too much time.*
♡ *It has to make me look and feel good.*

That is what this physical section is about: using exercise in a way you can enjoy and that makes you feel good in every way possible.

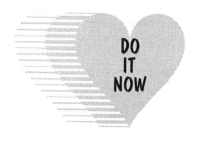

The first step is to find something you can enjoy doing. If your friend tells you what an excellent exercise swimming is, and you hate to swim, then swimming is *not* an excellent exercise for you. Find something you can like, or to begin with, at least not completely loathe. The possibilities for exercise are vast.

If you are currently doing no exercise, begin by committing to 5 - 10 minutes three times per week. Write it on your calendar as an appointment with yourself. Honor that commitment just as devoutly as you would a doctor's appointment or a visit to your hair stylist. These exercise appointments with yourself are just as important, and probably more so.

Exercise Tips:

☞ **Check with your health professional** before beginning a new exercise program.

☞ **Wear shoes appropriate to your chosen activity.** They should fit comfortably, giving your feet support, cushioning and protection. (Shoes do not necessarily require a designer label or the endorsement of a sports celebrity in order to achieve these humble objectives.)

☞ **Warm up** before engaging in the full exertion of an exercise, raising your body temperature a few degrees with slow, easy movements. This warms muscles and joints, reducing the chance of injury.

☞ **Keep your exertion at a level proper for your degree of fitness.** If you're not breaking a sweat by the end of your workout, you may need to increase your exertion a bit. If you can't converse without gasping, slow down. **If you feel tired, dizzy, or in pain, stop immediately!**

☞ **Cool down.** Reduce intensity by slowing your movements for the last part of your workout. This lets your body make a gradual shift to normal breathing and heart rate without "slamming on the brakes".

Aim to ultimately achieve 30 minutes of exercise 3 times per week or 20 minutes 4 times. Why not just exercise for 80 to 90 minutes one day per week and get it over with, you ask? If you are just beginning to exercise, it would probably hurt you. Also, the benefits of exercise start to reverse after 72 hours, so you would be back to Square One every time. It's essentially the same reason you don't brush your teeth for 45 minutes once a week.

There are now huge amounts of exercise information out there that will tell you to do some aerobic activity for the heart and lungs along with some resistance/weight training to build muscle. You can find the best ways to burn fat, tone muscles, live longer, go faster. . . . This is all wonderful, valuable stuff to know; but right now your mission is simply to get started, and to do it safely.

Walking is a great place to start. When you get a friend to join you, it can be even more fun and makes the time pass quickly. Move briskly! Your pace is just right if you can exchange scandalous tidbits without gasping from the exertion, yet still break a sweat.

Another possible choice is dancing to music at home. It does not require any special equipment, you do not have to dress up (although you can) and you are free to move and express yourself without fear of judgement.

Exercise can be important in crafting the body you want. It is not a singular cure-all, but as this book has continued to point out, it is one of many factors in being a whole, healthy person with a whole, healthy, attractive body.

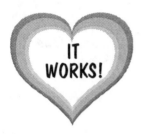

Why exercise is important for you:

1. It helps you look great! Exercise improves your circulation, and that means those red blood cells are whipping through your body like some E Ticket ride, bringing oxygen and nutrients to every cell in your body. (Besides being necessary to life, oxygen is an element critical to burning fat.) The blood cells are also carrying out the trash faster, so your cells (and thus your entire body) do not resemble some littered roadside.

2. Exercise makes you feel great! It stimulates the production of endorphins. Endorphins are your body's natural, no-side-effects drug that makes you feel euphoric when you are in love or when you open the Christmas present you always wanted—or when you exercise consistently.

3. Proper exercise makes your heart and lungs work a little harder and more efficiently. That makes them (you) a smoother-running machine and more resistant to disease.

4. I have done my best to avoid the "C" word—but exercise burns Calories. It burns them while you exercise, and also maintains an elevated metabolic rate that burns more for several hours after you stop.

5. A heightened sense of well-being and keener mental alertness are typical gifts of exercise. (Your brain is one of the recipients of the oxygen and nutrients.)

6. Many people find the time they spend exercising is generously returned to them in lowered sleep requirements, plus more mental alertness and productivity in their daily performance.

As with meditation, don't expect huge moving changes in your life after the first two sessions of dancing to your favorite music. However, you will definitely notice the positive effects of consistent exercise over time.

A Partial List of Exercise Activities

Aerobics
Funk
High Impact
Jazzercize
Low Impact
Step

Dancing
Ballroom
Ballet
Break
Country
Disco
Jazz
Tap

Hockey
Field
Ice
Street

Rowing
Canoeing
Kayaking
Machine

**Racquet
Sports**
Racquetball
Squash
Tennis

Martial Arts
Karate
Tae Kwon Do
Tai Chi
Aikido
Judo
Kung Fu

Skating
Ice
In Line
Roller

Skiing
Water
X-Country
Downhill

Baseball
Basketball
Biking
Calisthenics
Hiking
Isometrics

Nordic Track
Rope Jumping
Running
Soccer
Softball
Stair Climbing

Swimming
Volleyball
Walking
Wallyball
Weight Lifting
Yoga

EXERCISE

WEEK 1:

Date: _____ Type chosen: _____ Minutes:_____

Date: _____ Type chosen: _____ Minutes:_____

Date: _____ Type chosen: _____ Minutes:_____

WEEK 2:

Date: _____ Type chosen: _____ Minutes:_____

Date: _____ Type chosen: _____ Minutes:_____

Date: _____ Type chosen: _____ Minutes:_____

WEEK 3:

Date: _____ Type chosen: _____ Minutes:_____

Date: _____ Type chosen: _____ Minutes:_____

Date: _____ Type chosen: _____ Minutes:_____

Level Four Bodycraft Recap

After working with Level Four Bodycraft Tools for at least three weeks, are you:

Emotional: ♡ Looking into the mirror to love and affirm your body and yourself at least once daily?

♡ Creating a permanent emotional environment that attracts and supports your Bodycraft goals?

♡ Using your Emotions Journal daily and reclaiming the Rage to Live?

♡ Tapping the power of hidden emotions with the use of dominant/non-dominant hand dialogue?

Spiritual: ♡ Blessing everything you put into your body?

♡ Using affirmations to reshape beliefs?

♡ Finding the perspective of meditation?

♡ Seeking the support you need from others?

Mental: ♡ Reviewing your described body image goals every day?

♡ Indulging yourself with the fun and productivity of focused daydreaming?

♡ Treasure mapping?

♡ Reclaiming your mind-body voice?

Physical: ♡ Gradually increasing your daily water intake up to 1/2-ounce per pound of body weight?

♡ Eating more fruits, vegetables and grains?

♡ Breathing fully?

♡ Discovering that exercise and fun really can co-exist?

Before continuing to Level Five, examine your comfort level with each of these tools. If you are experiencing resistance or discomfort with any of them, you may want to focus additional time in that area, allowing it to become more workable for you. If the resistance or discomfort is extreme, let that part go for now.

When the Bodycraft Tools of Level Four feel like a normal part of your life-style, it's time for Level Five.

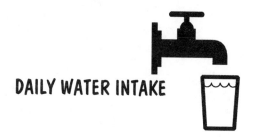

DAILY WATER INTAKE

Day 1_____   Day 8_____   Day 15_____

Day 2_____   Day 9_____   Day 16_____

Day 3_____   Day 10_____   Day 17_____

Day 4_____   Day 11_____   Day 18_____

Day 5_____   Day 12_____   Day 19_____

Day 6_____   Day 13_____   Day 20_____

Day 7_____   Day 14_____   Day 21_____

Your refrigerator is a good place to post this.

LEVEL FOUR NOTES

Note here any thoughts, ideas or resistance you experience.

What is working for you?

What parts make you feel good?

. . . MORE LEVEL FOUR NOTES

Fully relax, then ask yourself: "What do I most need to know or do right now?" (Use first your dominant and then your non-dominant hand to write any answers that may come to you.)

**AND JUST FOR YOU
. . . MORE NOTES**

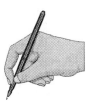

Level Five

Weeks 13–15

Chapter Eight

Bodycraft Tool #17: Fun (Emotional)

God respects me when I work, but loves me when I sing.

-Jewish Proverb

In the worlds of recovery and popular psychology, there is frequent attention devoted to getting in touch with the Inner Child. The Inner Child is the part in every human which enters the world with wide-eyed fascination, thirst for adventure, and unbounded creativity. On the road to adulthood, that part is frequently ignored, trampled, and abandoned; but it doesn't go away. The Inner Child may go into hiding, but its effects are always there.

The full spectrum of Inner Child work is outside the scope of this book, but one aspect is so important I would be remiss not to mention it—FUN!

Fun is an attitude that pervades and brings joy to all we do. It also includes the activities we can look forward to with anticipation and excitement—those things in which we completely lose ourselves as we do them.

As our society has become engulfed in the work ethic, fun has become a lost art. At best we promise ourselves we will do those things we love "when we have time". *Now* is the time to bring fun back to the mainstream.

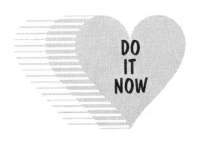

DO IT NOW

Have some kind of fun every day. If you're out of touch with fun in your life, you will first need to figure out what activities are fun for you. An exercise that can help you with this is to list every pleasurable, amusing or exciting thing you enjoy doing or think you would like to try. Use the following categories as guidelines:

♡ *Can do by myself*   ♡ *Do with other people*
♡ *Free or inexpensive*   ♡ *Costs money*
♡ *Spontaneous*   ♡ *Requires time to plan*

Having fun is a subjective, personal choice. Some people are thrilled at going to museums. Although that's an activity you may find pleasant, the little kid inside you might not jump up and down at the thought. When you choose an adventure for fun's sake, be sure it's something you can feel a bit giddy about.

Once you have these delightful, exciting activities committed to paper, the next step is to commit to doing at least one from each category. For the ones you can do immediately, do them. For those that require planning, get busy. Now.

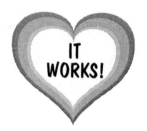

Why a daily dose of fun is good medicine:

1. It feels good.

2. It's part of a balanced life—often a missing piece that needs to be restored.

3.   Fun leads naturally to a happy state of mind. Scientific tests have repeatedly demonstrated that happiness promotes health, healing and long life.

4.   It keeps that Inner Kid happy. The alternative is an unhappy Inner Child which can be sneaky and vengeful if it isn't getting the "goodies" of fun. Some forms this internal revenge can take are general crankiness, illness, depression, accidents or even—AAUUGGHH!—weight gain! Makes you want to stop right here and go read the comics, doesn't it?

5.   Proverbs 15:15 states it the very best: "A merry heart hath a continual feast."

JUST FOR FUN...

❂ Laugh out loud.

❂ Read the comics and throw away (recycle) the rest of the newspaper.

❂ Invite friends over for breakfast, requiring that they wear their pajamas or bathrobes.

❂ For one day smile and say "hello" to every person you pass.

❂ Write yourself a letter about all your wonderful qualities (you know—the ones you keep waiting for other people to appreciate). Mail it.

❂ Spend a weekend in your own city pretending you are in a foreign country. (Even the most mundane corner grocery takes on a sense of the exotic.)

❂ Dare a kid to a water balloon fight.

Bodycraft Tool #18: Forgiveness and Grace (Spiritual)

Forgiveness is the key to action and freedom.

-Hannah Arendt

As you have already discovered, Bodycraft is not a program about losing weight (too easy to find it again), but rather a system which helps you let go of what isn't working for you in order to reclaim your individual perfection. Similarly, forgiveness—also known as grace—is a system which allows you to release what doesn't work so you can get on with the business of what does.

Some sources such as *Course In Miracles* and Louise Hay cite most body problems as stemming from lack of forgiveness. It is among the most powerful of healing tools, and when it seems impossible is when it is at its mightiest.

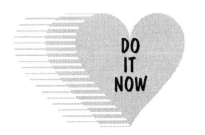

DO
IT
NOW

Examine the areas in your life where you are holding grudges or re-sentiments. Open your-self to the possibility of forgiveness in those areas. At first glance this may seem incompatible with the Emotions Journal. How can the same person furiously write about emotions, crush innocent ice cubes with a hammer, and do primal screams while mattress-bashing, without being a hypocrite about forgiveness?

Although it initially seems like a contradiction, the Emotions Journal is in fact a bridge to, and can be a major part of, the forgiveness process.

It is difficult, if not impossible, to forgive a person or situation when the emotion around it hasn't been fully discharged. The Emotions Journal, while helping you feel your joy, also lets you move through painful feelings such as anger, fear, and hurt so they can run their full course. At that point, and not before, they are ready to be released (forgiven).

The Emotions Journal/forgiveness connection is a two-way street. By opening to the possibility of forgiveness at the same time you are liberating your emotions, you can make the shift more quickly to grace.

Forgiveness doesn't mean condoning injustice or bad behavior. It does not come from the victim stance of, "It's okay that you burned my car and kicked my dog." Some things are not okay and never will be. What it does say is that you have learned all you can from the experience, and you are ready to let it go so it doesn't continue hanging around, sapping your energy, and clouding your passion for life.

Some people feel that by hanging on to their resentments, they are somehow punishing the "wrongdoers". Just as acid eats the vessel that contains it, resentment only makes life hard for the person who holds it.

Forgiveness is hardest to do when needed the most. The act of forgiving usually doesn't happen all at once but rather in small increments; and the first step is a willingness to forgive. Write or say it. "I may not feel like forgiving _____, but I am open to the possibility." That's all it takes to get started.

Inevitably, the hardest person to forgive is yourself. If you're feeling blocked about forgiving someone else, you are probably just as upset at yourself. Remember to frequently fill in the "I forgive _____" blank with your own name. Forgive yourself often, whether you think you've made a minor mistake or a world-class blunder. Forgiving yourself does not mean you've done something wrong or bad. It's a simple way of taking out the garbage and getting rid of even the smallest misperceptions of your goodness.

Another affirmation you can speak or write is, "I forgive _____ for not meeting my expectations." If you continue repeating it, even if you don't feel the least bit forgiving, it will start having its effect of releasing you.

(Remember, you're doing this for yourself. Is holding on to your favorite grudge important enough to also preserve a body image you would rather change?)

Keep repeating your commitment to forgiveness each day until you feel a shift. You will know when this shift is happening as you begin to experience a feeling of lightness inside.

Grudges and resentments are like ugly barnacles that can get attached before you know it. To stop them before they form, start the forgiveness process quickly. When you start mentally criticizing or judging someone (including yourself), immediately seek the comfort of grace. "I forgive you for not meeting my expectations." *You* will be the winner.

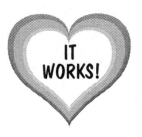

Why forgiveness is the most "graceful" tool in the Bodycraft process:

1. Forgiveness or grace bestows the gift of releasing the heavy, ungainly baggage that has been weighing you down both figuratively and literally.

2. Forgiveness clears out the debris of grudges and resentments that have been taking up your valuable space, time and energy. This makes room for all the good that has been trying to come into your life.

3. Anything in your life that isn't working is fair game for grace. It's not so much asking pardon as stating your readiness for release and freedom.

Without forgiveness, life is governed by an endless cycle of resentment and retaliation.

-Roberto Assagioli

Bodycraft Tool #19: Scales Are For Fish (Mental)

Bathroom scale down on the floor
Say I've dropped a pound or more.
I'm up another ten, you say?
You s.o.b., you've ruined my day.

You're standing on that bathroom scale again? Get outta here! Torture was long ago outlawed by the Geneva Convention, so stop it now! Every time you climb onto the Scales of Injustice, you are asking them to judge you based on a random number. "I'm stepping on the scale now. Am I a good person? Am I worth the air I breathe? Can I feel proud and happy today?"

If you have a problem with body image, the scale is not your friend. You have been giving your power away to an indifferent machine, letting it determine your thought process which affects your self-esteem and life path. If it's telling you all the numbers you love to hear, that gives you every reason to eat to a Full Tank. Right?

On the other hand, if the scales say your weight it up, then you certainly need to comfort yourself with a food toot after which you will feel doubly unhappy. This nasty dictator, for which you undoubtedly paid good money, is the Saddam Hussein of your household.

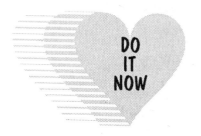

**DO
IT
NOW**

GET IT OUT! Get your bathroom scale out of your house this minute. And do not stop to weigh yourself "just one last time for old times' sake".

BODYCRAFT multi-purpose tip to get rid of this hideous contraption, return to it a small measure of the misery it has dealt you, and recoup some of your original investment:

Sell raffle tickets to slam-dunk the evil scale out a second-story window.

Most people think the scale is all that stands between them and physically ballooning into oblivion, the last control before losing all control. The truth is, it keeps you stuck. It keeps you in a mentality of judging yourself and asking others (even mindless machines) to judge you. It lets magazine articles intimidate you when they tell you how much (or how little) runway models and movie stars weigh, then encourages you to compare yourself to these people you don't even know based on that meaningless collection of numbered pounds. Knowing your weight does absolutely nothing to serve you in creating the body you want.

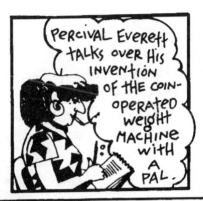

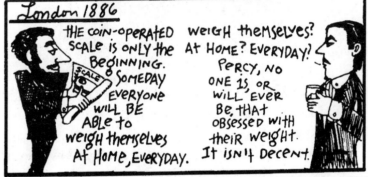

The bathroom scale is more addictive than the food that may have originally sent you there. If you are even now thinking of every reason you could never give up checking your weight, you're hooked. Think of being weighed as a prescription drug—it should only happen in your doctor's office. So get off it, you junky!

"How can I ever get the body I want if I don't know how much I weigh?" Since you are reading this book, I have to assume that knowing your weight has not worked great body magic for you up to now. Just when do you expect it to start?

The very best measure of your body is your body. How do you feel? If you are full of energy and feel happy, you and your body are at top performance. Congratulations! However, if you're missing the mark and feel blah, examine what tools you need for a tune-up.

For those who insist on a more quantitative measuring gadget, a full-length mirror is your best friend. Look at yourself in the mirror. (Do some mirror work while you're at it.) Is this how you want your body to look, or do you need to do some Bodycrafting? There. You have your answer, and it doesn't compare or judge you. It does not make you an unworthy person if you decide you want to make some modifications. It simply tells you what you need to know.

The next best measure is your clothing. How does it fit? If it's too tight, you either need to buy clothes that are more comfortable or trim a bit.

"How do I feel? How do I look? Am I comfortable?" Those are the three basic questions that replace the bathroom scale; and, unlike the scale, they give a much more truthful description of your relationship to your body. You are consulting your most valuable source of information—yourself. And these methods are not only more valid, but much more effective than any pound report.

The hardest part is learning to trust yourself. You really do know the truth, and you really can be trusted to do the best thing for yourself.

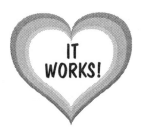

Why the bathroom scale should go the way of whalebone corsets:

1. Once you overcome the withdrawal from addictively jumping onto the scale, you'll be much happier. The symptoms and results are similar to getting out of any bad relationship.

2. Weighing yourself is not only useless but also counterproductive to creating the body you want.

3. Evaluating your body based on how it feels and looks as well as your overall comfort level allows you to start from a foundation of truth. Using your own powers of observation puts you directly in touch with your body instead of using the scale as a

middleman, while giving you a more exact idea of what kind of Bodycrafting modifications you want to make.

4. Getting rid of your scale is one more step towards getting away from negative self-judgment.

Bodycraft Tool #20: Posture (Physical)

Get your feet off the furniture. Brush your teeth.
Stand up straight.
  -Words to live by from Mothers Around the World

Up until now, you have been told to expect slow, gradual and long-lasting results as you Bodycraft. Here, for a change of pace, is a Bodycraft tool that gives the *immediate* results of improving your appearance, making you look 5-10 pounds thinner and contributing to your health. What is truly incredible about this is that it falls under the category of a "Mom-ism"— those universal truths that all mothers state on a regular basis and that kids refer to as nagging.

Clean your room. Wipe your feet. Do your home-work. Eat your vegetables. STAND UP STRAIGHT.

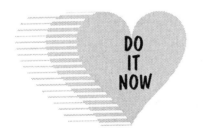

Ponder the amazing possibility that Mom was right this time, and consider all the benefits good posture holds for you. First look at any magazine advertisement featuring miraculous weight-loss "before" and "after" pictures. Typically the primary difference—besides that in the "after" photo they may have air-brushed half of the person's body away—is the posture.

In the "before" picture the subject is standing with a slouch, an exaggerated S-curved back, a protruding gut and a permanent glower. In the miracle of happily ever "after", the convert is standing tall and proud, back gracefully erect, stomach pulled in and face smiling. Such advertisements are much greater testimonials for the transformative effects of good posture than for mail-ordered, over-priced pills with terrible side effects.

Posture is not the only answer, but as with each of the Bodycraft Tools, it is part of the answer. It certainly provides a simple and effective kick-start for boosting not only your body image but your entire appearance.

Good posture entails somewhat more than just "standing up straight" in a rigid military position. Correct posture won't leave you in pain or unable to breathe. In fact, your proper body position should allow you to breathe freely, move efficiently, and improve your body's general performance.

If mothers were more technically correct, they would change their "Stand up straight" Mom-ism to "Stand erect." The back (or the spine, if your prefer) is the key to good posture, and in its natural healthy state is not perfectly straight. Looking at good posture from a side view, there is a slight inward curve at the neck, a slight outward curve of the upper back and another slight inward curve at the lower back.

To do a quick self-evaluation of your posture, stand facing a full-length mirror. Ideally, your head is straight and not tilted, right and left shoulders are at the same level (one should not be higher than the other), ditto for hips. Your knees and ankles face squarely ahead. A side view of your alignment (you may need an extra mirror, or have a friend snap an instant photo) should show your chin parallel to the floor; your ears, shoulders, hips, knees and ankles in a vertical line; and your back erect with its gentle curves properly aligned.

For professional expertise in evaluating and improving your posture, see a licensed physical therapist. You can find them in the Yellow Pages or get a referral from your doctor.

The American Physical Therapy Association has created a comprehensive brochure giving a physical therapist's view of posture. The brochure provides evaluations, suggestions and exercises in lay terms, accompanied by clear illustrations. At the time of this printing, the brochure could be obtained free by sending a stamped, self-addressed envelope to:

American Physical Therapy Association
"Posture"
Box 37257
Washington, DC 20013

Here are two exercises from the APTA brochure. They appear lengthy, but it will take you longer to read than to do them (about 10 seconds, repeated three times). The first is in a standing position and serves to improve or maintain good posture:

☞ *Stand with your back against a wall, heels about three inches from the wall and feet about six inches apart; weight should be evenly distributed.*

☞ *Place arms at your sides, palms forward.*

☞ *Keep ankles straight and kneecaps facing front.*

☞ *Keep your lower back close to the wall.*

☞ *Straighten the upper back, lifting the chest and bringing the shoulders back against the wall.*

☞ *Bring head back to touch the wall while keeping the chin tucked in as if a string is attached to the middle of the back of your head pulling it back.*

☞ *Pull up and in with the muscles in the lower abdomen, trying to flatten the abdomen.*

☞ *Hold position for about 10 seconds, breathing normally.*

☞ *Relax and repeat three to four times.*

☞ *Repeat entire exercise at least three times a day for optimum results.*

The following exercise, also from the APTA brochure, is for the lower abdominal muscles. Besides being effective, it is much easier than sit-ups and healthier for the back.

☞ *Stand comfortably.*

☞ *Clasp your hands and cup them around your lower abdomen.*

☞ *Pull up and in with the lower abdominal muscles, drawing in the abdomen.*

(This step isolates and strengthens the abdominal muscles. To locate the right muscles it might help to think of hiding your tummy under your chest.)

☞ *Hold for about 10 seconds.*

☞ *Relax and repeat four to five times.*

☞ *Repeat entire exercise at least three times a day.*

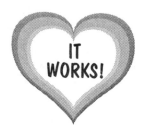

Some of the benefits of maintaining good posture and carrying it with you everywhere:

1. You look better. A lot better. Immediately. By carrying yourself in a way which lengthens and aligns your entire structure, you immediately appear thinner, with greater poise and confidence.

2. Glowing health is fostered as good posture properly aligns the bones which prevents undue stress on the joints, muscles and ligaments. The vital organs are in better position for their full functioning. Stomach muscles are strengthened, which in turn gives better back support. All of this contributes to a higher energy level and more bounce to the ounce in your muscles.

3. Your mother will be so pleased that you finally took her advice.

❦

Level Five Bodycraft Recap

After working with Level Five Bodycraft Tools for at least three weeks, are you:

Emotional: ♡ Looking into the mirror to love and affirm your body and yourself at least once daily?

♡ Creating a permanent emotional environment that attracts and supports your Bodycraft goals?

♡ Using your Emotions Journal daily and reclaiming the Rage to Live?

♡ Tapping the power of hidden emotions with the use of dominant/non-dominant hand dialogue?

♡ Having fun?

Spiritual: ♡ Blessing everything you put into your body?

♡ Using affirmations to reshape beliefs?

♡ Finding the perspective of meditation?

♡ Seeking the support you need from others?

♡ Using the release of forgiveness?

Mental: ♡ Reviewing your described body image goals every day?

♡ Indulging yourself with the fun and productivity of focused daydreaming?

♡ Treasure mapping?

♡ Reclaiming your mind-body voice?

♡ Abandoning your bathroom scale?

Physical: ♡ Gradually increasing your daily water intake up to 1/2-ounce per pound of body weight?

♡ Eating more fruits, vegetables and grains?

♡ Breathing fully?

♡ Discovering that exercise and fun can co-exist?

♡ Enjoying the immediate results of practicing and using good posture?

❦

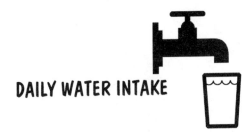

DAILY WATER INTAKE

Day 1_____   Day 8_____   Day 15_____

Day 2_____   Day 9_____   Day 16_____

Day 3_____   Day 10_____   Day 17_____

Day 4_____   Day 11_____   Day 18_____

Day 5_____   Day 12_____   Day 19_____

Day 6_____   Day 13_____   Day 20_____

Day 7_____   Day 14_____   Day 21_____

Your refrigerator is a good place to post this.

EXERCISE

WEEK 1:
Date: _____ Type chosen: _____ Minutes:_____

Date: _____ Type chosen: _____ Minutes:_____

Date: _____ Type chosen: _____ Minutes:_____

WEEK 2:
Date: _____ Type chosen: _____ Minutes:_____

Date: _____ Type chosen: _____ Minutes:_____

Date: _____ Type chosen: _____ Minutes:_____

WEEK 3:
Date: _____ Type chosen: _____ Minutes:_____

Date: _____ Type chosen: _____ Minutes:_____

Date: _____ Type chosen: _____ Minutes:_____

LEVEL FIVE NOTES

Note here any thoughts, ideas or resistance you experience.

What is working for you?

What parts make you feel good?

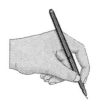

...MORE LEVEL FIVE NOTES

Fully relax, then ask yourself: "What do I most need to know or do right now?" (Use first your dominant and then your non-dominant hand to write any answers that may come to you.)

AND JUST FOR YOU
            ...MORE NOTES

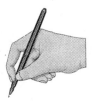

Chapter Nine

Coping With Positive Change

Every moment of your life is pivotal, allowing you to choose who you will be from that moment forward.

By using Bodycraft, you are creating transformation in your life. In many respects, you are assuming a new identity and leaving the old one behind, and that can create some uncomfortable feelings. This chapter addresses the different reactions you may notice in yourself and others as your goals and dreams become your personal success story.

As you reach your goals, you may begin to experience an inner battle of returning to self-destructive patterns while fighting to maintain the newer positive ones. Sometimes there is a feeling of uncertainty about who this new person in the different body is, and what happened to the other person who used to live here anyway?

If you start feeling conflicted about your habits or identity, disoriented, or stressed in ways relating to your Bodycraft success:

♡ *Evaluate the changes you have made/are making.*

♡ *Have a "meeting" of the former and the new self. Tell the old self how grateful you are for the many things it did to support and nourish you. It was that self who got you to achieve the changes that put it out of a job. Love it. Realize that the "former person" is still a real and positive part of who you are now.*

♡ *Grieve. You have lost something/someone, even though the loss represents something positive to you. It's seldom easy to let go of what we know and what is comfortable.*

♡ *Celebrate the new life you have crafted.*

You may need to repeat this processing on a periodic basis.

Your changing may be uncomfortable for some people who would much prefer to maintain their security by keeping you the same. Some may not even know what they're reacting to. If you start feeling resistance from others (or even from yourself):

♡ *Reaffirm your desires for yourself and why you desire them.*

♡ *Reaffirm your worth and your right to be the person you most want to be.*

♡ *Remember your opinion of yourself is among your most valuable assets.*

♡ *Remind yourself that you are the owner of your body and your life. In spite of the messages given by the media and perhaps even family and friends, your appearance and what you do with it are your own business.*

♡ *This is an excellent time to keep reviewing your goal statements from Level One (Bodycraft Tool #3) on a daily basis.*

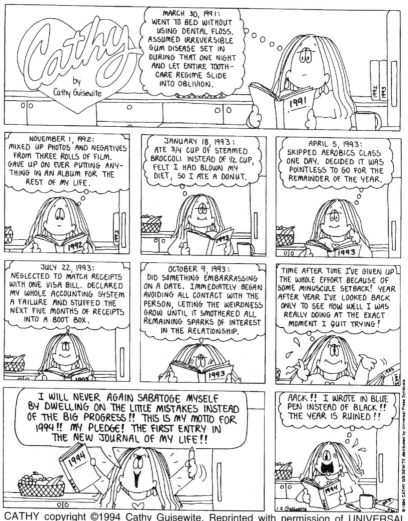

Perfection Paralysis

Perfectionism gives birth to Procrastination. Together these notorious thieves rob us of creativity, esteem and accomplishment.

What if. . .oh no, this is just too horrible a thought to even entertain. But, well, what if you don't do Bodycraft perfectly?

What if on the second day or third week or during the Fourth Level or at any time you don't use all the tools, or don't use them completely or even quit doing the whole Bodycraft process for awhile? What's a body to do?

If you're still interested in doing it and have found that it has value for you, then do it. Do it in a way that you can live with.

Who ever went whiz-bang from Ground Zero to Perfection when learning a skill or crafting new abilities? With most new projects we have to learn from our stumbling blocks until we achieve proficiency. And even proficient isn't perfect.

If you've put yourself on a time table, stop it. You have forever to do this, assuming you choose to do it at all. Bodycraft is not designed to make you miserable, but rather to comfort and support you.

Start over. Or start in the middle. Just do it. Do it as imperfectly as works for you.

Don't allow an over-honed sense of perfection to keep you from getting what you want. All-or-nothing usually ends up with nothing. Be courageous enough to embrace mediocrity if need be. "Mediocre" has become such a taboo concept, but it wins hands-down over Perfection Paralysis.

Our past is not our potential.

Goals and Dreams—a Package Deal?

All rising to great places is by a winding stair.
-Francis Bacon

If you have unconsciously pinned all your hopes and dreams on having your ideal body shape ("Everything in my life will be perfect once I have a beautiful body."), it can be scary to reach that goal without the benefit of the mansion, the relationship, the luxury car, the loving family, the exotic travel or whatever you had envisioned to go along with it.

What happens when the dreamed-for body starts to happen and all the other hopes and dreams are not automatically there with it? It may seem easier to sabotage the slender body and return to hoping and dreaming rather than facing that you still have most of the same problems and the fears. You just get to face them with a body that can run up a flight of stairs without wheezing and doesn't make waistbands chafe.

To avoid any self-sabotage that could occur at this point, look at the hopes and dreams that go along with the great body. When you're visualizing your desired body, what other expectations go along with it? Recognize them and write them down as separate goals. Make plans to achieve those individually rather than expecting a package deal.

Bring what might be hidden dreams into consciousness—get into the real world and look at each step you need to take to make each goal happen. Dream, but remember to stay anchored in the reality of doing the step you need to do today.

The following is a brief exercise to examine the whole package of dreams and goals and what you can do to make them a reality.

When I think about crafting my ideal body, what is the whole package I think of with it? What dreams do I have that go along with looking the way I have always wanted to look?

What are the goals I need to achieve those dreams?

What steps can I take to achieve the goals?

What are my fears? [This is also a good time to write in your Emotions Journal.]

What is the worst case?

What is the reality?

What is the very best case?

What do I think will actually occur?

What am I willing to do to make it happen?

Bodycraft won't fulfill your every ambition, nor will it automatically produce your dream romance. The odds of it picking a winning lottery number for you are about the same as for Madonna calling you to request etiquette advice. What Bodycraft *will* do is show you how to make your dreams of a beautiful body a physical reality and add some balance to other aspects of your life. With that, you have the tools to go forward and do the rest yourself.

Chapter Ten

The Journey Continues

Too low they build, who build beneath the stars.
-Edward Young

You have been given 20 tools (plus a few nuts and bolts) to put into your living toolbox. Like a hammer, a rake, a shovel or screwdriver, they only work if they're taken out and used. Nothing was ever created with tools that stayed in a drawer—except maybe dust.

At the beginning I mentioned my journey continues. Through the years of processing and seeking, these tools have become integrated as a part of me. I find it's still possible, however, for some of them to slip into disuse.

If your experiences are like mine, there may be times when your body image is out of kilter, when you start gaining a few pounds, or when you aren't nurturing yourself and quit paying attention to your basic needs. Sometimes even when the mirror says otherwise, you may feel fat. Regardless of how that feeling of discomfort presents itself, it acts as a clear message to examine those tools you need to dust off and actively use.

Your perceptions and your body will change quickly when you focus on these processes. Once you have set them back into motion, it's possible to let them continue functioning on their own with little conscious effort.

As you experience the personal success that comes with making Bodycraft part of your lifestyle, you may wish to investigate more ways to enhance your body and your life. Here are a few additional thoughts.

Life Giving Touch

Babies, even with the most nutritious food, can't survive without touch. Even as adults, we die a little—or maybe a lot—without the nurturing of physical touch.

Hugs are one of the best ways to give and receive the miracle of touch. If you aren't comfortable hugging or being touched (and this is a strong indication you need the nurturing it can provide), start with someone who is very close to you. This could be a friend, parent, spouse, daughter or son. If you can even touch that person on the hand, that's a start. (It goes without saying to only touch and be touched by those with whom you feel safe.)

Hug yourself! Wrap your arms around you, and say, "I love you." It sounds as corny as being in a Disneyland parade wearing a silver medal, but it feels terrific.

Massage is another touching way to exchange energy. If you're trading massages with a friend and are not comfortable with a full body massage, try a hand or foot massage. Shoulders also love the attention of touch. If you opt for a professional massage, ask friends to recommend a Certified Massage Therapist.

Being In Your Body

"Well, gee, where else would I be?" you may ask. Surprisingly, most of us spend a lot of time not being in our bodies. As children many of us learned to avoid trauma by detaching and "going somewhere else". It may have been a good survival tool that served us well at the time, but it's probably not beneficial now and could actually be a detriment.

I have discovered that when I have vague feelings of uneasiness, being at loose ends, or a sense of unfulfillment (such as those times when I'm standing in front of the refrigerator for too long), I'm not fully present in my body. At such times I usually need to deal with something I may not be acknowledging, and this is one method of escape. Sometimes I may be just "floating" out of old habits.

The best antidote is to first become fully conscious of your body and to ground yourself. Imagine your torso as a tree trunk and the root system running down through your legs. Visualize the roots continuing on down your feet, deep into the ground. You are now a solid part of Mother Earth. Imagine taking nutrients, comfort and support gladly provided by the Earth into those roots and absorbing them into your body. Feel your body and the energy rising in it. Feel your toes, feet, legs, buttocks, stomach, torso, chest, shoulders, arms, hands, fingers, neck and head. Feel every part of your body individually and as a whole. Feel yourself grounded, whole and fully present in the moment.

Consider Vegetarianism

Vegans use no animal products at all. Ovo-lacto vegetarians include eggs and dairy products in their diet. This is not a move to be made quickly or without thought, but there are many benefits to vegetarianism making it worth examining as an alternative.

A vegetarian diet typically has a lower fat and cholesterol content than one including meat, and usually translates to a healthier, thinner body. (The reason I qualify this statement with "typically" and "usually" is because it is possible to prove this isn't always the case by consuming large amounts of cheese, nuts or other highly concentrated sources of fat.)

Vegetarian consumption is also easier on the planet. This is not the place for a forum on ecology and animal rights, but getting in just one quick plug: a vegetarian diet is a step in the right direction for both—not to mention for your own personal ecology.

Should you choose to pursue this, I recommend you begin by gradually reducing and eventually eliminating red meat. As you are doing this, increase your consumption of legumes (beans, lentils, garbanzos), grains and vegetables. Then begin reducing and eliminating poultry from your diet and, finally, fish.

There are now hundreds of excellent vegetarian cookbooks available. There are also hundreds of bad ones, so be sure to thumb through before purchase. My personal favorite is *Nikki & David Goldbeck's American Wholefoods Cuisine: Over 1300 Meatless Wholesome Recipes from Short Order to Gourmet.* (They also get my award for Cookbook With the Longest Title.) I find their incredible array of recipes to be clear, easy to prepare and delicious. Try them.

Examine Excess

This is another of those issues requiring a delicate balance. One of my favorite axioms is: Moderation in all things—including moderation. (Or, excess is fine as long as you don't overdo it!) I believe life is to be gulped and not sipped, but it's important to make sure we aren't choking on it.

You are invited to examine any excesses choking your life including but not limited to: caffeine, sugar, alcohol, nicotine, (whether or not you care about the health effects of smoking, can you shrug off the fact that it gives you wrinkles and makes you smell gross?) chocolate, and fat.

If after careful consideration you decide you would like to do with less of some things, think of how you can replace what you are limiting. It may be a similar but more wholesome consumable; it may be a thought or idea. Do you need to cater to some of your other senses—sense of smell, touch, hearing, vision? Are there small luxuries with which you could nurture each of these? Only you will know what is appropriate for you.

I enjoy my coffee and tea. In fact, I have never found a caffeine molecule I didn't adore. When I find myself consuming too much coffee and overeating due to caffeine-induced hunger, experiencing skin break-outs, whirring around like a ceiling fan and generally being uncomfortably "amped" with a caffeine buzz, I know I'm consuming addictively and want to make some changes.

If I were to tell myself to give up or even reduce caffeine, I would probably rebel and drink more. Instead, as I start thinking of a great cup of coffee, I replace it with the thought of radiant health and skin, feeling great, and being powered with real, not synthetic energy. I will usually then have a cup of juice or water or herb tea. It feels satisfying because I'm not giving up anything but instead am making a different and gratifying choice.

Looking at your personal areas of concern, decide what choices you can live happily with that will best serve you for the long term.

❦

Epilogue

This book was written over a long period of time and for a number of reasons. I first started writing down these tools and experiences because I needed a clear road map for myself when the path got hazy. But as I started organizing my many scraps of paper and putting scribbled notes into a coherent order, the strongest motivation became a desire for people like you to share the path with me.

Thank you for taking part in making my dream a reality and for joining me on this exciting journey of self-discovery. As I have learned to love myself, I extend that love to you.

I welcome your letters, comments, suggestions and success stories. Please send them to:

Ilizabethe Zélandais
c/o Anti-Gravity Press
P. O. Box 348002
Sacramento, CA 95834-8002

I look forward to hearing from you.

Appendix A

Any Twelve Step program, and in this case Over-eaters Anonymous specifically, can be an effective means for putting your life in order. The Twelve Steps vary somewhat from program to program, but for the most part create a level playing field for living life. This is a valuable gift for anyone who was not reared with clear, consistent, loving guidelines for creating a clear, consistent, loving life or lifestyle.

Seldom, if ever, will any of us be in 100% accord with an institution, group or another individual. Even with the respect and loyalty I have for OA and other Twelve Step programs, there are some of their precepts with which I disagree.

My first difference of opinion deals with the accepted introduction when someone shares. "Hi. My name is Jane. I am a(n) _____." Fill in the blank with "compulsive overeater", "alcoholic", "addict", or whatever addiction is operative for that individual or particular program. It is immaterial the individual may have been in active recovery for 20 years. I respect the reasoning for this: it breaks down denial, and also serves as a reminder that a compulsion or addiction may be in remission but is not gone. My objection to that format is that "I am" is the strongest affirmation one can claim for anything whether positive or negative; and I do not want to keep reclaiming my addiction.

The second issue arising is the reluctance of OA or AA to allow the Twelve Steps to be altered. Again, this is understandable in the light of maintaining a powerful structure that works, and not having the Steps diluted or distorted. However, I find some of the phrasing in the Steps to be unacceptable. So I have adapted my own Twelve Steps.

I would encourage you to fully explore the Twelve Step Programs exactly as they are and make your own decisions based on claiming your own power. There is even a phrase in Twelve Step Programs appropriate to this: "Take what you need, and leave the rest."

The Adapted Twelve Steps

1. I am powerless to control people, place and things. When I think I can control them and attempt to, my life becomes unworkable.

2. I focus on myself and the Higher Power dwelling within me, and my life has focus and peace.

3. I make a decision to create and live the life I want by opening myself and my life to the guidance of my Higher Power.

4. I thoroughly, honestly and lovingly seek an understanding of who I am, including my strengths and weaknesses.

5. With my Higher Power and another person, I examine the fears, limiting beliefs and negative thoughts in my life. I also look at my courage, unlimited ways of being and my positive attributes.

6. I accept the integration of my wholeness and the willingness of my Higher Power to remove the fears, limiting beliefs, negative thoughts, people, places and things that no longer work in my life.

7. I ask my Higher Power for guidance and strength in making changes within myself and my life for the highest good of all concerned.

8. I make a list of everyone I have harmed, and I am willing correct each situation. I make amends to heal myself and others, and I clear up unfinished business. I forgive myself and others for all mistakes and injuries. I bless us all.

9. I make a list of everyone whose life I have touched in a positive way, and I open myself to those blessings.

10. I live consciously, treating myself and others lovingly, accepting opportunities for growth, constantly seeking and expecting the highest good for myself and others.

11. Through such gifts as prayer, meditation and fun, I open my awareness to the wonders of Life and my Higher Power.

12. I practice these steps every day, and change them as I find even higher ways of living. I allow my life to be a transforming presence everywhere I go, just because I AM.

❧

Appendix B

My experience with meditation while visualizing the color spectrum—red, orange, yellow, green, blue, indigo, purple and white—has had some additional benefits.

I used to be sensitive to lack of full spectrum light—i.e., inadequate sunshine. When it rained or was overcast for more than one or two days, I would become depressed and irritable. After about six months of using color meditations, I noticed overcast days had very little effect on my emotions. My assumption is that with the meditation, I created my own internal source of full spectrum light.

If you become depressed on cloudy days, this meditation might be worth a try. It costs nothing, has no harmful side effects, and takes only a small amount of time. It's also highly portable.

Another similar meditation involves focusing each color on the associated chakra. Chakras are energy centers located along the spine. The first chakra (red) is located at the base of the spine and is associated with security. The second (orange) is right below the navel and is associated with sexuality, creativity, play and delight. The third (yellow) is at the solar plexus and is associated with use of the will and synthesis of the emotions. The fourth (green) is at the heart level and is associated with love, healing, new growth and transformation. The fifth (blue) at the throat is associated with all types of communication and self-expression, power and peace. The sixth chakra (indigo) is located between the eyebrows or "third eye" and is the area of clairvoyance and use of the sixth sense as well as inner knowing. The seventh (purple) at the top of the head or crown is associated with highest good, higher knowledge and higher purpose. The eighth (white) starts about a foot above the head and is associated with the Higher Self.

When I meditate using the colors in conjunction with the chakras, I do it the same as the "hall" meditation, except the light is emanating from the chakra then expands to surround my body.

Resources

Bach, George R. and Goldberg, Herb. *Creative Aggression: The Art of Assertive Living.* New York: NAL/Dutton, 1993.

Bell, Lorna, R.N. and Seyfer, Eudora. *Gentle Yoga.* Cedar Rapids, IA: Igram Press, 1982.

Bradshaw, John. *Homecoming: Reclaiming and Championing Your Inner Child.* New York: Bantam Books, 1990.

Brennan, Barbara Ann. *Hands of Light.* New York: Bantam Books, 1988.

Capacchione, Lucia; Strohecker, James; Johnson, Elizabeth. *Lighten Up Your Body, Lighten Up Your Life.* North Hollywood, CA: Newcastle Publishing Co., Inc., 1990.

Carlson, Richard. *Everything I Eat Makes Me Thin.* Bantam Books: New York, 1991.

Chopich, Erika and Paul, Margaret. *Healing Your Aloneness.* San Francisco: Harper & Row, Publishers, Inc., 1990.

Dossey, Larry. *Healing Words: The Power of Prayer and the Practice of Medicine.* San Francisco: HarperSanFrancisco, 1993.

Gawain, Shakti. *Creative Visualization.* New York: Bantam Books, 1982.

_____. *Living in the Light.* Mill Valley, CA: Whatever Publishing Inc., 1986.

Goldbeck, Nikki and Goldbeck, David. *Nikki & David Goldbeck's American Wholefoods Cuisine: Over 1300 Meatless Wholesome Recipes from Short Order to Gourmet.* New York: Plume, 1984.

Groger, Molly. *Eating Awareness Training.* New York: Summit Books, 1983.

Hay, Louise L. *You Can Heal Your Life.* Santa Monica, CA: Hay House, Inc., 1984.

The Holy Bible. King James Version. Cleveland, OH: The World Publishing Company.

Keep Coming Back. Center City, MN: Hazleden Foundation, 1988.

Kent, Howard. *Yoga for the Disabled.* Wellingborough, Northamptonshire, Great Britain: 1985.

Kirschmann, John D., editor. *Nutrition Almanac. 3rd ed.* New York: McGraw-Hill Book Co., 1990.

Packard, Joan. *Natural Breast Enlargement Through Effective Relaxation Techniques.* Sacramento, CA: Jalmar Press, 1981.

Pearsall, Paul. *Making Miracles.* New York: Prentice Hall Press, 1991.

Prudden, Suzy. *MetaFitness: Your Thoughts Taking Shape.* Santa Monica, CA: Hay House, 1989.

Ray, Sondra. *The Only Diet There is.* Berkeley, CA: Celestial Arts, 1981.

The Spindrift Papers. Lansdale, PA: Spindrift, Inc., 1993.

Stearn, Jess. *Yoga, Youth, and Reincarnation.* New York: Doubleday & Company, Inc., 1965.